UNDERSTANDING DISEASE

A Health Practitioner's Handbook

John Ball

BLACKDOWN PUBLICATIONS

BLACKBOROUGH, CULLOMPTON, DEVON EX15 2HH

First published in Great Britain in 1987
by Blackdown Publications

© John Ball 1987

Typeset by Exe Valley Dataset Ltd., Exeter
Printed by SRP, Exeter

British Library Cataloguing in Publication Data

Ball, John B.
. Understanding Disease: A Health Practitioner's Handbook
    1. Pathology   2. Therapeutic Systems
    I. Title
    616   RB112

ISBN 0-9512559-0-8

Contents

To Gabrielle, with love

Foreword

Culled from his training and experience in orthodox practice (Dr Ball was a GP from 1970–81), and also from teaching at various schools and colleges of complementary medicine, the author has written a book which addresses the former from the standpoint of the requirements of the latter. Its primary purpose is to describe pathological processes in the language of orthodoxy while offering explanations in simple and clarifying terms. It is a book of immense utility. Those who have come to health care through a route other than medical school will appreciate the value of a systematic analysis of disease, and through familiarity with the language of pathology be able to communicate with their medical colleagues. There is no doubt in my mind that there are only gains to be made out of bringing these two apparently disparate approaches into communion. The process is, I believe, similar to any 'marriage of opposites', a necessary step in the direction of wholeness and maturity.

The medical doctor, traditionally observing the tenets of his Hippocratic Oath, is not permitted to divulge medical knowledge. The times are changing in this respect as well as in respect of acknowledging the limitations of this system of medicine. The treatment which it offers is often suppressive, usually productive of iatrogenic side-effects and leads to various long term though often unacknowledged consequences.

The premise upon which most forms of complementary medicine stand is that the symptoms are the language by which the diseased organism finds expression. They are the outward evidence of the internal disorder, providing the healer/physician with a true guide, like Dante's Virgil, a lead into the hidden interior wherein the disturbance is centered. Furthermore, the symptoms are understood to represent the best possible adaptation which the organism can muster in order to save itself from a deeper, more permanent and more destructive form of disturbance. From this point of view it is self evident that any form of treatment which suppresses the symptoms will inevitably lead to the eventual intensification of the suffering. However, this conclusion is usually not drawn because it is assumed that the disease is an entity in itself, a unique syndrome of symptoms, independant of the sufferer and therefore dealt with as if it were an enemy – attacked and destroyed. This view closes the mind to further possibilities, because once the symptoms have been extinguished it is deemed *a priori* that the disease has been vanquished. Another reason for the lack of a true interpretation of the disease is due to the habit of compartmentalising the information which is received from the patient. Spirit, emotions, mind and body are each treated as though separate; even the physical body is subdivided and specialists consulted whose role is to examine, diagnose and eventually treat the parts.

Practitioners of complementary medicine tend to emphasise a synthetic and embracing philosophy of healing; it is because of this bias that they need to pay particular attention to the paradigm of Western medicine, itself an outcome of the reductionist and causal model of reality. This model is powerful because the manipulation of concepts leads to mastery of matter. However, mind may be divorced from feeling in the interest of expediency. This unilateral view is responsible for much mischief, for feeling associates while reason isolates. Suffering is a common concomitant of civilisation; its alleviation may be sought through an awareness of soul processes and the reconnection to the spiritual heart, the feeling centre of our life's purpose. Having made this statement it must nonetheless be borne in mind that the great insights of science may be used for the benefit of man, no less in the field of healing. Medical science, with its store of observation, the accumulated evidence of centuries of recording and correlation, contains testimony to both the miracle of life and the tragedy of disease. It is a description of the physical field within which we find ourselves. Unlike the treatment which is offered on the basis of dubious premises, the description of the body and the pathology it is heir to cannot be refuted.

Misha Norland. June 1987.

Preface

This book has evolved from several years of lecturing and discussing the often controversial topic of disease with homoeopaths, osteopaths, herbalists, acupuncturists and other healing professionals. Each of these disciplines has its own map of the human mind and body, and the ills which befall them, and most recognise that all attempts to construct a single all-encompassing model describing the human condition is impossible, so an understanding of different viewpoints is needed for the complete picture. Indeed the resurgence of interest in alternative methods of pursuing health is largely due to the emphasis which science has placed on disease processes, to the point where the patient and his or her suffering has been supplanted.

Any realistic approach to illness must include an objective appraisal of the dysfunction of the body (pathology), an understanding of how the patient sees the problem (empathy) and a philosophy of diagnosis and treatment which may involve a wide range of perspectives and skills. What follows is an attempt to walk a tightrope between knowledge and understanding, so that the science of pathology and all its clinical manifestations becomes comprehensible without the dubious necessity of surrounding oneself with a fortification of information for its own sake, which is as able to erect barriers as destroy them. Hence the book is hopefully not a catalogue of diseases but an appraisal of the disorders likely to be seen in the average working life of a practitioner. Rare diseases hold the same sort of fascination for medical authors as rare birds do for birdwatchers and most medical texts give a disproportionate amount of consideration to once-in-a-lifetime problems. This may mean that some readers will feel short-changed by the absence of parathyroid disorders for example, but the line has to be drawn somewhere and those conditions affecting less than 1 in 20,000 of the population have been ignored or only mentioned in passing.

If the core of medical science is understood the patient with a rare disease can be pursued in standard texts.

An understanding of the structure and function of the human body has been assumed, there is not enough space to include anatomy and physiology, nor more than a brief description of orthodox treatment. Medical terminology has been used where relevant, not because it is strictly necessary but rather because without a minimal understanding of the terms a student is unable to refer elsewhere nor a practitioner to explain the jargon to patients. As the majority of words are of Greek or Latin origin the translation is given for clarity and interest and a glossary of terms appended at the back. This includes a number of words which are not in common usage today but appear in some of the classic texts of homoeopathy, and are so labelled.

Textbooks of medical science make depressing reading for those susceptible to suggestion, and many students may imagine themselves to be harbouring all manner of ills as they turn these pages. All I can say to them is that it probably isn't what you think and you probably won't get what you imagine!

My thanks are due especially to my friends Misha Norland and Tim Fox who have made many helpful suggestions about the contents, and to Donald, my father, who has ironed out many of the hiccoughs in the course of the book. Also to Dr Keith Ball for his pertinent comments on the chapters on the the heart and vessels. Clare Yerbury as given some very useful advice about the graphics, as has Richard Kelly who also designed the cover. I have also been greatly aided by Colin Tucker of Exe Valley Dataset Ltd who has gone to great lengths to advise with the typesetting.

I

Health, Pathology and Disease

The prevailing attitude of the majority of people today is the Cartesian one, that the world in general and the body in particular are the sum of their parts and can be dissected, analysed and adjusted to perform better. Orthodox medicine in fact looks on the body as a machine, and this is both its success and its failure. The failure of orthodoxy is its apparent inability to distinguish between the body and the person, and in making the assumption that they are identical. This is the inevitable consequence of the convergent, analytical approach based on specialisation, where increasing technology allows us to focus on ever smaller details of the 'machine' at the expense of the 'owner'. The success of orthodoxy lies in its refusal to be distracted from measurement, so that it has developed refined and logical techniques for describing, categorising, diagnosing and in some cases treating disease.

We are now moving, it seems, into a post-Cartesian era which can encompass other models of the body. The reason for the move appears to be two-fold, firstly the realisation by science itself that matter is relative, and secondly the willingness to embrace other belief systems as disillusionment with materialism increases – more and more of the same does not appear to be the solution. It is becoming apparent that the only way forward is to examine the whole ecological framework within which a 'disease' prospers and find ways of adjusting that environment so that the condition simply evaporates with the course of time. Indeed the model we are left with is that of the body as a continually changing process kept in dynamic equilibrium by its own internal gyroscopes. In short we are back to the Taoist philsophy of the 4th century BC.

It may be that patients understand this intuitively when they turn away from the academic citadels and seek out 'alternative' medicine. It may be that more and more practitioners sense this as they opt for alternative or complementary methods of healing, but whatever is the case it seems that what Werbach calls 'Third Line Medicine' is here to stay, and we are left finally with the realisation that a single model cannot encompass the huge intricacies of the human being and that circumstances alone can dictate our methods. This is not to say that there will be no need for the doctrine of specific causes, that would be to throw the baby out with the bathwater, but persistence with a single conceptual approach is likely to become less useful with time.

Health

Although most of this book is concerned with diseases, we should perhaps start by looking at what constitutes health. This is not easy to define as everyone has their own concept of an ideal body with no physical, emotional or mental discomfort and a pervading sense of well-being and fitness. In purely physical terms health is a stable internal environment maintained in the face of external changes to which we have learned to adapt in the course of evolution. That is not to say that the adaptive process is always comfortable, in fact it is this very discomfort which we call 'suffering', but that is not the same as illness. What one individual will take in his or her stride may cause another great suffering, for one of the greatest barriers to health is not so much the illness itself but the emotional reaction to it. It is precisely because we have come to assume that science can provide a cure for every situation that we are now in a state of suffering, because our mind is so full of unfulfilled expectations.

The chronic effects of stress, pollution, faulty diet or unhappiness are subtle and do not begin to make themselves felt until the chain breaks at its weakest link and pathology shows itself in one form or another. Just to look at this pathology in isolation is to examine a single slice of a continuum of events, and it is important to realise that the same stimulus has been affecting other aspects of the body which may only later fail. Therefore to try and reverse that particular disclosure of the body without looking beyond is of limited benefit, although it may be worth doing.

It is certainly quite often the case that the physical aspects of disease, i.e. the pathology, can be influenced in some way by the scientific approach, but in most cases the physical manifestation is only the final expression of a process which has been continuing for a long time. What we have come to consider in the post-Cartesian era are the events which lead up to that change, and these events are usually in the realm of a different model.

The Era of Tolerance

If pathology is the final expression of a provocation then we should perhaps be spending more time looking at the events leading up to the disease, rather than examining the disease itself. This may seem obvious and much has been written about the way in which our National Health Service has become a National Disease Service (Brian Inglis: The Diseases of Civilisation), but one of the main reasons why scant attention has been paid to prevention is because it is neither easily measurable nor very predictable.

If we look at the era which precedes the outbreak of pathology, the duration when external stimuli are apparently tolerated with impunity, we see no visible reaction, no measurable consequences. All that can be measured are the stimuli themselves, and as the Cartesian approach is to discard what cannot be quantified any idea that the body could be influenced by a 'self regulating tendency' within itself is also discarded as mere speculation. As is the possibility that as well as being disrupted by events the 'tendency' (for want of a better word) may fluctuate of its own accord and even be amenable to treatment.

To translate this into a three dimensional model as in Fig. 1.1 the Cartesian view will be from above, in which case nothing will appear to happen until the sudden emergence of a pathological state from below, and subsequent bodily changes. The direction and rate of change together constitute the shape which the pathology and therefore the disease takes, and this change can be opposed by a variety of methods, principally drugs and surgery.

Most complementary practitioners, however, view events in the model from the side, and therefore see something rather different. They must, of course, formulate some concept to explain what occurs in the 'era of tolerance' before the

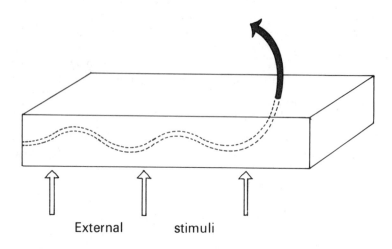

External   stimuli

Fig. 1.1   *The era of tolerance and the emergence of pathology*

emergence of symptoms, and a wide variety of names have been given by various cultures from the Classical times onwards. These include *Ch'i, the vital force, prana, the subtle body* and even the *aura,* and while there are those who would dispute the similarity between these terms most of these disputes have more to do with the methods used to influence the direction of this 'force' than with the force itself.

Because the era of tolerance has not so far proved amenable to methods of objective study (Kirlian photography may be an exception to this), it has largely been dismissed as fanciful by scientists. And because any changes which take place are subjective they are generally felt by someone who is in a relatively undistracted state. This crucial fact leads to the curious and rather amusing situation that those who are distracted by seeking for objective evidence do not, by and large, experience it due to their very distraction. While those who engage in such meditative practices as enable them to catch glimpses of it develop a fascination which tempts them to abandon measurement and even spurn it as unnecessary. It is these disparate views of the same situation which has created the two camps of health practice today, with their tendency to mutual repulsion.

Expressions of Pathology

When we use the word 'disease' we usually think of a recurring pattern of change found in certain people, often those of a similar age and sex, which is manifested either as subjective symptoms or as objective changes in the body. It mostly happens that the symptoms occur first – as pains, weakness, itching, tremor, disorientation, faintness etc, and only much later, if at all, do detectable changes happen to the body. Pathology is the name given to the study of changes in the tissues which result from some form of inadequacy of adaptation, and it is this study which forms the cornerstone of orthodox medicine.

The reasons why our adaptive mechanism fails may be inherent in our make up, or due to overwhelming challenge by some stimulus or another, and these types of failure account for the varieties of congenital and acute diseases. The majority of chronic illness is more complex than this, however, and is a combination of predisposition, inadequate defence and repeatedly maintained challenges in the form of nutrition, radiation etc. Faced with this the body has a variety of standard ways of expressing its discomfort, and these constitute the main varieties of pathology outlined below.

The experience of patients subjected to these forms of pathology will differ to some extent depending on the organs involved, the rapidity of onset and even their age, and it is these differences which account for the varieties of symptoms in any disease. In general the law of probability applies in that the unusual symptoms of common conditions are far more likely to occur than the common manifestations of rare diseases. As far as diagnosis is concerned it is important to be able to work backwards as well, and use symptoms as a way of excluding possible underlying pathology – remember that the commonest reason for missing a diagnosis is the fact that the possibility never crossed your mind. In this connection it is important to ask oneself what likely pathology could be encountered in a person of this age and sex and then ask specific questions at some point to unearth the necessary information.

Inflammation

The standard response of the body to sudden challenge from

heat, light, radiation, chemicals and organisms is inflammation, characterised by the classical symptoms of *pain, heat, swelling* and *redness*. For inflammation to occur there must be a reaction in the local blood vessels, and this takes the form of dilation (causing redness and heat), followed by an increase in their permeability (causing the pain and swelling). This enables the phagocytes, those white cells responsible for engulfing foreign bodies, to migrate through the wall into the tissues, as well as the plasma proteins with their antibodies and clotting factors. The way in which the inflammatory reaction is quickly brought about is by the liberation of *histamine* and other chemicals, especially from the mast cells but also from others. Following this the reaction may quickly subside with minimal pain felt as itching (as in nettle stings), or be continued indefinitely as chronic inflammation by a group of chemicals first discovered in the prostate gland and therefore known as the *prostaglandins*.

Inflammation of one kind or another is seen in the majority of acute diseases, and swift resolution usually follows. If the inflammatory response is inadequate a much more prolonged situation may occur, as may be observed in such conditions as TB, syphilis, rheumatoid arthritis and Crohn's disease. The normal phagocytes of the blood, the polymorphs, are unable to do the job and hand it over to rather more specialised cells, the macrophages ('big eaters') which are modified monocytes which have left the blood stream and settled down to a long life in the tissues. There they can engulf very large particles but produce large quantities of fibrous tissue which swells up to look like a tumour, so these swellings were given the name *granuloma* by the early pathologists and are the characteristic feature of many chronic diseases.

The way in which the inflammatory response manifests and resolves is reflected in the symptoms of many diseases, particularly those classified as infections. In some there is complete and rapid resolution and such conditions as mumps and measles therefore run a predictable course. In others there may be areas of suppuration where the tissues break down and result in abscesses (collections of pus), ulcers and later scarring. Sometimes the organisms penetrate the containing tissues and invade the lymphatics or blood vessels to cause septicaemia and profound toxaemia. In general the more specialised a tissue is the less it is able to regenerate after being inflamed, so that connective tissue such as bone will usually heal successfully but such tissues as nerves, kidney and muscle will not.

Tumours

In most people's minds the word 'tumour' is synonymous with cancer, and this is a grave error in thinking, for the literal meaning is simply 'swelling'. Since we are composed of cells, and each of those cells has the ability to divide about 50 times in the course of our lifetime before the process grinds to a halt, it is highly likely that this process of division, or mitosis, may under certain circumstances become distorted to a greater or lesser extent. Normally any abnormal cells will be eradicated by the immune system as if they were foreign to the body (see chapter 3), but if the changes are minimal then they may only be detectable under the microscope.

Two terms are applied to such minimal changes, the first being *metaplasia* which refers to a reversible change from a fairly complex cell into a more simple one such as may occur on the cervix, and is the first indication that something is amiss. If the change proceeds to alteration in the size and shape of the cell then the term *dysplasia* is used and this is less likely to return to normal. Understandably, both types of altered growth are the result of prolonged minor trauma and may if untreated become progressively abnormal culminating in a total escape from control.

Once this escape has occurred, *neoplasia* or 'new growth' is said to have happened and the coded instructions which the genes relay to the new cells become corrupted, leaving the cell to continue dividing but with no control over when to stop or how to differentiate into specialised tissue. If the former alone occurs then the neoplasia is said to be benign and the new cells may push aside their neighbours and cause symptoms due to pressure but will not invade or infiltrate other tissues nor *metastasise* to distant sites. Moreover the plethora of new cells will look very similar to their parents and closely resemble the tissue of origin.

But neoplasia is not always benign and if the cells are sufficiently damaged, for instance by *carcinogens* (cancer-producing substances), then the offspring will revert to primitive forms which do not differentiate into their specialised tissues and are thus said to be *undifferentiated* to a greater or lesser degree. In general the less differentiated a neoplasm is the greater its degree of malignancy and vice versa. We can see then that the difference between a well differentiated malignant tumour and a benign tumour may be very slight and barely discernible under the microscope except by an experienced pathologist yet this is of great significance when the question of surgery arises.

Tumours are labelled according to their tissue of origin, and this may be epithelial tissue (mucus membrane or skin), glandular or connective tissue of one kind or another. Benign epithelial tumours look like smooth warts and may even have a small stalk so are termed *papillomas* (L. papilla = nipple). Because the epithelial surfaces of the body are most likely to come into contact with carcinogens many of the malignant tumours arise here and are known as *carcinomas* (Gr. carcinos = crab), and are usually prefixed by their tissue type, e.g. 'squamous cell carcinoma of bronchus', 'transitional cell carcinoma of bladder'.

Benign glandular tumours tend to arise in endocrine glands where they may lead to some of the malfunctions described in chapter 16 on hormonal disorders, and they are termed *adenomas* to distinguish them from the malignant *adenocarcinomas* (of which the commonest example is the breast). Connective tissue tumours which arise in fat, muscle, cartilage etc are common and almost always benign – for instance fibroids which are seen in the smooth muscle of the uterus, lipomas which may appear as soft fatty lumps under the skin. They are generally given the name of the tissue in which they arise with the suffix *-oma*, such as fibroma, chondroma, osteoma. However on the few occasions where the connective tissues do produce malignant tumours, they are among the most malignant known and tend to arise in younger people. They are given the suffix *-sarcoma*, e.g. osteosarcoma, fibrosarcoma etc., after the Greek word 'sarx' meaning 'flesh'.

Degeneration

However much care we take of our bodies it is unfortunately a fact that they start to degenerate at a certain stage and although we can slow this process up we cannot reverse it to any great extent. This deterioration which we know as ageing starts at around 30–40 and is nature's way of ensuring that a large percentage of a single species does not continue to exist beyond reproductive age as this reduces the possibilities for the more vigorous members, a fact which some of us are unwilling to take to heart(!). Fortunately human (male) society has been able to arrange things so that accumulated experience continues to dominate where physical prowess long since fled the stage, but in this respect we are unusual in the animal kingdom.

It is rather ironic that degeneration often takes place most rapidly in those on whom the environment appears to lay least stress, and this is largely a modern phenomenon. A diet so rich in refined carbohydrate and saturated fat coupled with little need to use the calories has resulted in new forms of nutritional pathology such as diabetes and atheroma to replace those of rickets and 'chlorosis' as iron deficiency was once termed.

One can postulate two types of degenerative change, one based on the above over-accumulation of metabolites in cells which are unable to discard them either because of excessive quantities or equally due to abnormal chemicals in the form of food additives and pollutants. Such changes may be tolerable in cells which are renewing themselves periodically, but once our body arrives at a point when it is composed of cells which are no longer actively dividing but can only deteriorate, then the accumulated excesses will exert rapid changes on a variety of organs.

It is at this point that the osmotic pressure of the surrounding fluid will overwhelm the delicate pumping mechanism of the cell which will flood with water and swell. It is here that the accumulated fatty deposits in the walls of the vessels will obstruct the passage of blood and oxygen and lead to anoxia of the tissues. And it is now that our previously supple cartilage will become fixed with deposits of calcium salts in a vain attempt to strengthen weakening fibres. But ultimately we must all succumb to the failure of whichever organ we have, knowingly or unknowingly, abused the most, and by doing so begun the unravelling of the web which knitted together sustains our life.

2

Allergy: Disorders of Ecology

Nature has no interest in the survival of the human race. At least, no more so than any of the other species. She functions as the great balancer, a sort of free economy where different groups ebb and flow according to conditions. For millenia this is how life functioned and harmony reigned, until humans identified themselves as the most important of all the species, which must have been around the time when we started breeding animals for food, instead of hunting them and being hunted on equal terms. It still took a number of centuries for us to develop tools of sufficient destructive power to upset the balance of nature, but finally by the mid 20th century the stage was set. Pesticides and fertilizers ensured sufficient food, antibiotics and hygiene a longer life and the population exploded, leaving a trail of ecological damage which may take an equally long time to repair itself. In the late 20th century we are hopefully beginning to reverse the damage done not only to the environment but to ourselves as well. Great interest has arisen particularly in the fields of immunology and allergic disorders, and in the way in which our bodies react to pollution of all types. The name for this new approach is *clinical ecology*.

The Immune System

Our natural ability to withstand outside interference from micro-organisms is assisted by several defence mechanisms (defensive from our point of view at any rate), and the chief of these is the immune system. Under normal circumstances, when an organism or other foreign protein is found in the body it is immediately 'arrested' and taken to the local lymph node, where certain cells known as *B lymphocytes* set to work and in a few days produce an identical progeny or 'clone' of plasma cells which in turn produce proteins called *antibodies*. These antibodies are specially fashioned so that they key into the protein coat of the invader, which is termed an *antigen* as it generates antibodies. This type of 'lock and key' configuration is together known as an 'immune complex', and renders the organism harmless until it can be removed by phagocytes. In case there are more organisms on the way, many more antibody 'keys' are made and stored as *immunoglobulins* in the body, so that we are a warehouse of different types of antibody stored in readiness. This, of course, is the basis for most types of immunisation. Some organisms like tetanus and scarlet fever try to beat the system by secreting powerful poisons called toxins which damage the host, but lymphocytes can produce antibodies against these proteins too in the form of antitoxins. Because most of these antibodies are stored in the blood they are termed *humoral antibodies* to distinguish them from other, *cell-mediated*, antibodies which are located in the cells of the tissues.

There is a possible snag, however, which is that the B lymphocytes must be careful not to make antibodies against parts of their own body, which they have to recognise. This is done by having a pair of 'educated' *T lymphocytes* standing behind each B lymphocyte either helping it or suppressing it according to whether or not they recognise the protein (they are called T lymphocytes because they receive their 'education' at an early age in the thymus gland). If they are damaged (as happens in AIDS) or make a wrong decision then either no antibody gets made – immunodeficiency, or antibodies against the body's own tissues are formed – autoimmune diseases.

T lymphocytes also have another role to play, and as well as monitoring the activity of B lymphocytes they also produce a series of antibodies which do not circulate as immune complex in the blood stream but instead police the tissues as cell-mediated immunity. Their responsibility is to reject larger entities such as the large bacteria, fungi, cancerous cells and transplanted tissues, and because they take rather longer to act their reactions are known as *delayed hypersensitivity reactions*. A typical example of one of these is the Mantoux test for TB which takes several days to exhibit.

The earliest studies of the immune system were largely related to immunisation and vaccines, and it was only later that attention was switched to the phenomenon of allergy (Gr = other work) and hypersensitivity. This was something of a puzzle to investigators who had assumed that immune reactions could only benefit the host, but it seems that the system has evolved to over – rather than under – react and this is simply the price we have to pay for our defence. Indeed it is arguable that these reactions are always inappropriate, for they may be telling us that our body is uncomfortable with the way in which it is being treated.

Allergy

To understand this we need first to take a closer look at the immunoglobulins, those 'keys' made by the B lymphocytes. These come in five slightly different varieties or classes, each with a specific role to play, and each is therefore given a distinguishing letter. Starting with the most abundant the letters are G, A, M, D and E, and because they are all immunoglobulins these are abbreviated to IgG, IgA, IgM, IgD and IgE.

IgG forms the majority and circulates throughout the blood and tissues, even crossing the placenta. Along with IgM it forms the majority of the immune-complexes mentioned earlier. IgA is located especially in the secretions of the gut and has a role to play in hypersensitivity to foods (see next section). IgD does not appear to have been found a very significant role as yet, but it is IgE, the antibody which is least abundant, that causes the most allergic problems.

It has long been known that certain individuals react in a specific but unpleasant way each time they come into contact with certain substances – usually house dust, animal fur or pollen in the air – and so they were named *atopic* which means literally 'out of place'. Atopy runs in families and manifests clinically as asthma, hay fever and eczema, and it is known that atopic children have up to six times the normal amounts of IgE, located in the skin and mucus membranes. The actual cells in which IgE is found are called *mast cells*, and when stimulated they release large quantities of histamine and other similar chemicals very rapidly, which cause smooth muscle to contract and vessels to leak fluid in large quantities – the very symptoms of asthma and hay fever. This is one of the commonest and most studied of the hypersensitivity reactions, and is sometimes classified as *type 1 hypersensitivity*.

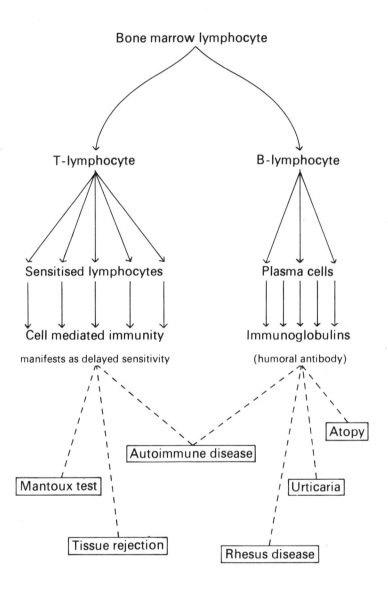

Fig. 2.1   *The mechanism and possible consequences of immunity*

In a few individuals the type 1 hypersensitivity is more widespread and they may suffer a sudden severe reaction after an injection of a foreign substance such as penicillin. There is collapse and difficulty breathing, with drop in blood pressure, a condition called *anaphylaxis* or anaphylactic shock (Gr = to ambush), and it is possible that this could be the explanation for some cases of 'cot death' in young babies, but in this case what is the means of introduction of the allergen, as no inoculation is evident?

It was noticed that the condition of *urticaria*, also called *hives* or *nettlerash*, happened in some after eating certain foods such as shellfish, strawberries, eggs or even the chemicals present in them as dyes or preservatives. This condition must operate through IgE as the reaction was so swift, often within half an hour or so, and produced the typical evidence of a histamine reaction with swelling, itching etc. Sometimes the reaction is general and all the tissues swell, most noticeably those of the eyelids and lips which are loosely bound – *angio-oedema*. Here, then, is a food allergy with all the ingredients for anaphylaxis present, moreover there is good evidence that cot death occurs around the time of weaning when new foods are being introduced and that it is more common in non breast fed babies. It was considered that allergy to cow's milk could be a cause, and this led to the speculation that food was more involved in the whole spectrum of illness than had been previously thought.

Food Intolerance

The reactions to some foods that we have just described are clear-cut and dramatic, even though the exact ingredient which triggers the reaction is not always obvious. In practice, however, many patients seek help for symptoms which do not fit clearly into a textbook picture of disease, symptoms like headache, catarrh, diarrhoea, distension, depression and a host of others. Or if they do fit into a disease category, such as ulcerative colitis or rheumatoid arthritis, it is one for which no clearcut cause has emerged, and some of these patients, though by no means all, respond dramatically to what is called an elimination diet.

What is the mechanism by which some foods appear to lead to these adverse reactions and why are they 'masked', i.e. delayed?

This question is at the core of the controversy over clinical ecology, and is not easily answered, in fact many scientists would argue that no connection can be made unless some test can show an objective reaction either by skin testing or changes in antibody levels in the blood or some other measurement such as hair analysis. Unfortunately the state of the art does not as yet permit a conclusive test, but even in the absence of one it seems as though orthodoxy is now becoming more impressed by the results of treatment which, like homoeopathy, are individual and thus not easily reproduceable on a large scale.

One possible explanation of the mode of action was first documented by physiologist Hans Selye in his work on stress adaptation. Selye described three stages which an animal goes through after physical, chemical or immunological stress. It first goes into a state of reaction in the form of some degree of shock, when adrenalin circulates, then within a variable time gradually adapts to the new circumstances, during which it is reliant on cortisone from the adrenal cortex, but finally exhausts itself and enters a phase of inability to adapt as the supplies of cortisone are exhausted. It is this final phase of exhaustion, often brought about by intervening disease, childbirth or trauma which often acts as the precipitating factor for symptoms which had previously been unexpressed. This would explain why foods which had been tolerated for years, even to the point of addiction, suddenly become noxious.

Such a scenario may even apply to babies who, at the moment of birth, are extremely vulnerable to infection and so are donated a large supply of IgG and IgA antibodies through the mother's milk. Because IgA particularly is contained in the secretions of the gut it may provoke a reaction to an antibody swallowed by the baby, and manifest as the all-too-familiar colic. This may happen after the baby is introduced to new foods, around the age of three months, or even occur whenever the breast-feeding mother has eaten a particular type of food.

If food intolerance is suspected then an elimination diet is recommended as the most direct means of establishing the connection, as it is seldom possible to tell from a dietary history alone. All food should be eliminated for a period of five days, and only mineral water permitted to drink. At the end of this time different foods should be reintroduced one at a time, preferably beginning with those which have been on the menu since homo sapiens came down from the trees, such as fruit and meat, and only introducing grains and dairy products later.

Susceptibility and the HLA system

The 'educated' T lymphocytes have an awesome responsibility in recognising whether or not a substance is foreign to the body, and subtle errors of judgement result in certain types of disease processes. To help them to keep track of which cells are of their own kind, most of the cells in the body are as it were 'stamped' with a particular configuration of proteins as an antigenic marker on the cell membrane. Thus each person has a unique set of markings (except for uni-ovular twins who share the same stamp) and as these were first discovered on the leucocytes they are known as the Human Leucocyte Antigens or *HLA system*. In order to produce this stamp one of the chromosomes in the cell nucleus sets aside four spaces (called A, B, C and D) on each of which a specific antigen is inscribed rather like the PIN number on a cashcard. This has two particularly significant consequences.

The first is in the field of susceptibility to disease. It has been noted that the sufferers of some conditions are likely to have a certain type of HLA antigen; thus people with psoriasis are likely to possess antigen number 6 at position C, so this is termed HLA C6. Similarly rheumatoid arthritis is associated with D4 and both diabetes (the juvenile onset variety) and coeliac disease with D3. In some diseases the association is only slight, but in others it approaches 100%; for instance 96% of patients with ankylosing spondylitis have HLA B27, and 85% of coeliacs D3. This does not mean that these antigens in any sense cause the disease, indeed there are many who have the relevant HLA antigen who never display symptoms, but it does give us a much better model for understanding the concept of susceptibility within a measureable framework. Another useful by-product of the presence of these antigens is their assistance in coming to a diagnosis, especially in the early stages of a disease when the symptoms may be unclear, as the presence or absence of an HLA antigen will be a significant pointer in one direction.

Another use of the knowledge of the HLA system is for the matching of organs and tissues before transplantation. Organ transplantation has only become possible hand in hand with advancing knowledge about immunology, and it seems that the closer the match of the HLA antigens on the four positions, the less likely rejection is to take place. Tissue-typing is now routinely performed and hopefully at least two and perhaps three of the four antigens can be matched – the key does not have to fit perfectly in the lock to turn it! As was said before, some tissues have more HLA antigen than others, consequently corneas are relatively easy to graft, kidneys moderately so, heart and lungs more difficult and the liver hardest of all.

Cancer

The body reacts to malignant tumours in its tissues in the same way as it does towards grafts, by rejecting them. It is able to do so because the healthy immune system recognises cancer cells by the abnormal antigens which they carry, called 'tumour specific antigens', which mark them out for destruction. The process of 'cancering' appears to be happening all the time as mutating cells throw up primitive forms at periodic intervals, but this is of little consequence as long as they are swiftly discovered and destroyed, and it is only when a defect in the immune system allows one of these potentially independant tissues to escape control that the 'disease' of cancer is said to have occurred. So it is obvious that cancer cannot be transmitted from one person to another by injecting them with malignant cells. Indeed, there are those who consider that the immune system in mammals developed primarily as a safeguard against these internal dangers rather than against threats from the environment in the form of micro-organisms.

A dramatic example of this occurred in 1968 in America when one of the early kidney transplants was being performed. Unbeknown to the surgeons the donor kidney contained a very early cancer and when a routine postoperative chest Xray was performed some weeks later the attendants were startled to see several rapidly enlarging secondaries. Surmising that these could only have come from the kidney, this was re-explored and found to indeed contain the primary tumour which had taken advantage of the immunosuppressive drugs used to prevent graft rejection. There was no alternative but to remove the donated kidney and stop the drugs, whereupon the lung secondaries rapidly regressed and the patient recovered.

Once a tumour has established itself, it may relentlessly go on to destroy the body but this is unusual. More commonly a balance is reached in favour of the tumour but the immunological mechanisms fight a rearguard action and slow its growth, sometimes even reversing it. The outcome largely depends upon the ability to revitalise the ailing immune system which allowed the tumour to occur in the first place. For this reason removing the primary site of growth may actually increase the rate of spread of secondary metastases because it was the primary tumour which was stimulating a reaction in the immune system. However, this is by no means always the case, and sometimes the secondaries regress or are slowed down.

The inability to eliminate colonies of malignant cells increases with age and hence we see a higher incidence of cancer in the elderly who tend to have an impairment of their cell-mediated immune system. We also see a higher incidence in those tissues and organs of the body which are exposed to a multiplicity of antigens during their lifetime and this may explain why the tissues of the lung, breast, stomach, colon, cervix and skin, which are in constant contact with potential allergens, are therefore more liable to cancer.

Immune defects

Such a complexity of operations is involved in the protection of the body that it is perhaps hardly surprising that one breaks down from time to time and we are left vulnerable to any passing micro-marauder. On rare occasions children are born with a defect in the system and no immunoglobulins are made, so that once the maternal antibodies are lost they rapidly die of infection at the age of six months. More commonly defects are acquired in the course of time, and until the arrival of the condition we call AIDS this was usually the result of tumours of either the lymphocytes or the plasma cells, and known as Hodgkin's disease or multiple myeloma respectively.

Hodgkin's disease is a form of cancer involving the T lymphocytes which are located in the lymph nodes and the spleen, and is seen mostly in teenagers and young adults, especially men. There is painless swelling of the glands in the neck and chest, and these small, rubbery swellings later enlarge to a considerable size and extend to the other lymph tissues. At the beginning of the disease there is sometimes a fluctuating fever every few days, with night sweats and sometimes a general itching of the skin. An unusual and very significant feature is pain in the bones or the glands coming on after drinking alcohol. With treatment the prognosis is very good and over 80% survive. A similar condition called *lymphoma* or 'non-Hodgkin's lymphoma' occurs in older people and is rather more malignant.

Multiple myeloma is a cancer seen mostly in the elderly and involves the *plasma cells* derived from B lymphocytes in the bone marrow, which produce huge numbers of a particular 'runaway clone'. These proliferating plasma cells are all of the same type and therefore manufacture vast amounts of the same IgG antibody, far more than the body requires. A large mass of plasma cells develops in the marrow and causes nagging, deep pain in the bone or else a spontaneous fracture. The cells metastasize and take over other sites in the marrow, so the skeleton becomes studded with multiple areas of cells which crowd out the other developing cells leading to anaemia, thromocytopenia (lack of thrombocytes) and neutropenia (lack of neutrophils). The result is the clinical symptoms of bruising and infection so characteristic of the disease, so that death from pneumonia is common. The blood is so overloaded with IgG from the plasma cells that it spills over into the urine but cannot be seen unless the urine is heated, when it precipitates in a cloud of 'Bence-Jones protein', only to redissolve on boiling.

AIDS

Fear, sex and righteous indignation are the preferred ingredients of a good headline as any journalist will tell you, and the condition of acquired immunodeficiency syndrome which we have come to know as AIDS has been billed for all three. It has come to occupy a corner of our mind previously reserved in the Victorian era for syphilis and in the middle ages for the Black Death. And all within the space of four years and a total death rate of 30,000, equivalent to that caused by smoking among the same population in 22 days! Why? The main reason for fear is the uncertainty which the condition causes, particularly exactly how it spreads and whether it will develop in someone infected, and if so how soon. These are all questions to which there are at present no certain answers, but in the seven years of its existence we have come to know quite a lot about it.

We know, for instance, that to date the increase has been almost completely exponential, doubling approximately every twelve months, and that it is likely to do this for at least several more years as cases come to light which were contracted prior to the much increased awareness about how the disease spreads. But after that it is almost certain to level off as awareness of the condition and its mode of transmission become more widespread, and it is largely a question of the speed of social and individual change which will curb the growth, otherwise the outlook is grim indeed. Nevertheless AIDS is a disease we are going to have to live with for a long time and may have some far-reaching social consequences. What follows is a brief summary of the facts as they are known hitherto.

The Epidemiology: Until 1985 the majority of sufferers were gay or bisexual men (76%), intravenous drug users (17%), haemophiliacs (1%) and others who had inadvertantly been given contaminated blood (2%). The remaining 7% were heterosexual men and women or children, some of whom had contracted the disease in utero. Since then there has been an upturn in the last group, consistant with expectations and indicating that there are a large number of symptomless carriers who are unknowingly able to spread the disease by heterosexual intercourse. It is among this latter group that the spread of AIDS is most likely to continue as sexual practices are unlikely to change very rapidly until, as in the gay population, friends and acquaitances contract the symptoms. By then the numbers possessing the virus will run into several hundred thousand, for it is estimated that for every patient exhibiting symptoms there are between 50–100 carriers of the virus. What is uncertain at present is the percentage of carriers who will go on to contract the disease, but the current estimate is 30% within 5 years.

The Agent. There is very good evidence that a virus is involved in AIDS, and this had been suspected from the beginning owing to the great similarity with some of the features of hepatitis B, especially related to the transmission by blood. Until 1985 this was unproven, but simultaneously a French and American team of researchers detected in the blood of an AIDS carrier a virus similar to that causing leukaemia in some races and found within T lymphocytes, so it became known as human T lymphocyte virus III or HTLV III (later changed to HIV or human immunovirus). The virus selectively damages the helper T lymphocytes so that the excess number of suppressor cells left effectively prevent the B lymphocyte from functioning and making antibody, leaving the body immunodeficient and exposed not only to infection but also to neoplasms. The virus is known to be present in blood, semen, saliva and breast milk, but has not been detected in urine or faeces. However the amount present in saliva is so small as to render contracting the disease from kissing virtually impossible, and it is also quickly inactivated by hot water or detergent.

The Symptoms. The manner in which AIDS first came to light was when a number of gay men developed an unusual type of *pneumonia* in which the protozoon *pneumocystis carinii* was implicated. This was strange because this parasite is normally quite unable to make inroads into the body except in transplant patients who are immunosuppressed with drugs. It was also found that other *opportunistic infections* were present, such as *herpes, Candida* and even TB in some. Another group were found to have a rare form of skin tumour – *Kaposi's sarcoma*, which raised livid dusky weals on the skin in various parts of the body. Those with opportunistic infections survived on average for about a year, while the prognosis for those with Kaposi's was nearly twice that long. About one third of the patients developed symptoms in the CNS, beginning with changes in mood and then progressing to stupor and finally *dementia*.

These patients had in fact been carrying the virus for a good many years before succumbing, and in retrospect the symptoms they noticed at the time when they first came into contact with the virus were fairly inocuous, amounting to a slight fever, sore throat, headache and diarrhoea for a few days which quickly passed and were dismissed as 'flu'. However, within six weeks or so the body will have made antibodies against the virus, a process known as 'seroconversion', and these may be detected by examining the blood in what has come to be called, rather misleadingly, the 'AIDS test'.

Pre-AIDS. In between contact and (perhaps) getting the disease a number of chronic problems may arise, and this is sometimes known as the 'pre-AIDS period'. These occur as the immune response weakens and there is therefore a persistant enlargement of the lymph nodes all over the body, especially in the neck and axilla, which may be present for many months or years–*persistant generalised lymphadenopathy*. If this then deteriorates into AIDS it is heralded usually by dysphagia from oral or oesophageal thrush, night sweats, weight loss, perianal ulceration or involvement with the nervous system.

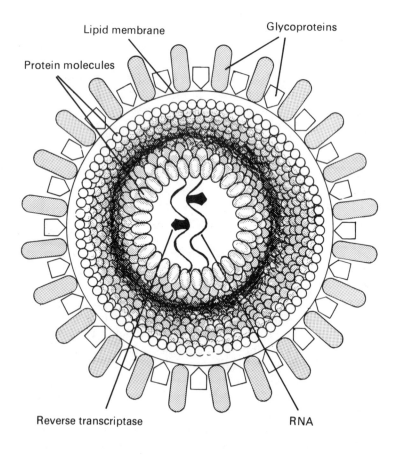

Fig. 2.2   *The AIDS virus*

Autoimmune disease

It was an early axiom of immunology that the body could never injure itself in any way and that the immune system was unable to turn against itself. All the evidence, however, indicates that on certain occasions it will do just that. In fact we have already seen how the tissues of the lungs and gut may at times over-react and lead to self-inflicted injury in the form of allergies, although these are in the main restricted to the surface of the body. It appears that under three separate circumstances the body engages in a form of civil war which expresses itself as one of the 'autoimmune diseases'.

The first of these, and the most common, is the group of organ specific autoimmune diseases in which cells from a secretory gland are disrupted for some reason and leak their contents into the blood. There they come into contact with the lymphocytes which read them as foreign, since they have previously been screened from any contact, and go on to make antibodies against them, and these can be detected by examining the blood. This antibody reaches the gland and sets about destroying it, so that eventually it atrophies and a deficiency disease results. The glands involved are the thyroid (Hashimoto's disease), the stomach lining (pernicious anaemia), the pancreatic beta-cells (insulin dependant diabetes), the hair follicles (alopecia), the salivary glands (Sjogren's syndrome) and many others.

The second situation is rare, affecting about one person in 20,000, and results in a condition called *systemic lupus erythematosis*, so-called because of the prominent red, saddle-shaped rash on the nose reminiscent of the stripe of a wolf (lupus = wolf). SLE had been known for years as a condition of young women leading to kidney failure, arthritis and other systemic malfunctions, but the cause remained a mystery until strange deposits of immune complexes were noticed in the kidneys and these were found eventually to be antibodies against the nuclear material of the body's own cells. It seems that normally the nuclei of cells are well hidden from the immune system, but on occasions break down to release large molecules of DNA which act as antibodies, and the ensuing immune complexes block any small vessels in the body and cause inflammation there, so the disease runs a prolonged course until kidney failure usually terminates matters.

A rather different type of autoimmunity occurs where the antigen of an invading organism happens to be identical to that of one of the host's own tissues, with the result that the antibody formed, having seen off the invader, then goes on to set about its own organs. Once again, it is the glomerulus of the kidney which is often selected, as well as the synovial membrane of the joints and the tissues of the heart. The results take the form of the diseases which are known as *acute nephritis* and *rheumatic fever* and are discussed in the relevant chapters.

3

Infection: Disorders of Susceptibility

The Concept of Infection

The Industrial Revolution which transformed Europe in the 17th and 18th centuries brought with it a series of epidemic diseases which swept into the overcrowded cities and ravaged the populations. These took the form of cholera, typhoid, smallpox, diphtheria and TB especially, and medical opinion was divided into three opposing theories about the cause of infectious disease – the contagionist, the miasmatic and the zymotic. The contagionists held that minute particles were spread through food and water, and that these multiplied in the body as 'animalcules'. The miasmatists felt that disease was the result of noxious gases which they called 'miasms' (although not quite the same as what Hahnemann meant when he referred to miasms), and that these arose from decaying matter. The zymotic theory considered that each infectious disease was the result of a specific ferment or 'zyme' and that they were passed by contact from one body to another. All the ideas had something of the truth, but were unable to shed any light upon prevention apart from the isolation of cases in quarantine for forty days (Fr. quarant = forty).

Into this arena came two men who were to change opinions, the German pathologist Virchow and the French bacteriologist Pasteur, and both were able to make use of the microscope which had been invented two centuries before by the Dutchman van Leeuwenhoek, but which had only recently been sufficiently developed to view what came to be known as 'microbes'. Virchow believed that all disease was fundamentally a result of cellular abnormality, and to that extent he is often considered the father of pathology. His view was that under normal circumstances the cells of the body are able to adapt to the changes which might in others lead to disease, and he emphasised susceptibility, believing that microbes were largely the by-product of disease rather than its cause, although he never denied their existence. Pasteur, however, was able to demonstrate the microbes and also to prevent the outbreak of certain diseases by the use of his vaccines, and the medical and pharmaceutical professions tended to his view rather than emphasising susceptibility and prevention. In fact most of the decrease in the infectious diseases were due to social, environmental and dietary improvements and took place before the advent of antibiotics and immunisation.

The Micro-organisms

Only a few of the vast numbers of the different types of micro-organisms are actually pathogenic, and the majority of these fall in the categories of viruses and bacteria. Larger than both of these, but still invisible to the naked eye, are the tiny protozoa (such as amoebas) and fungi which are also involved in certain disease processes. Much larger species than this, the insects and worms which infest rather than infect us, are easily seen with the naked eye and therefore not technically micro-organisms at all.

To compare the enormous range of size involved, let us assume the average human cell to be the size of a refrigerator. A red corpuscle will be as big as a car tyre, and a bacterium a football. Viruses will vary in size from a grape to a pea, depending on the type. In the other direction a protozoon will be the size of a packet of cornflakes or larger, while the multicellular organisms like lice and worms will be the size of a house.

Viruses

Because of their minute size (they are the smallest living creatures), viruses could not be visualised directly until the invention of the electron microscope in 1937, but long before this their existence had been assumed because of the ability of an unknown 'poison' (the Latin word for poison is 'virus') to pass through filters which remove bacteria. Finally some of the substance was crystallised and found to be composed partly of either RNA or DNA, the nucleic acids of which the genes in the nucleus of the cell are made. It was then realised that a virus reproduced by taking over the duplicating apparatus of the nucleus and substituting its own blueprint, so manufacturing its own kind and finally killing the cell. Because the essential ingredients of the virus were virtually identical to those of the host cells, this meant that any form of chemical destruction by the newly-invented antibiotics was out of the question and it was only the body's ability to form antibodies that prevented capitulation.

Viruses are involved in many of our commonest infectious diseases. The common cold has variable symptoms and may be a result of the activities of any of four different families of viruses, of which one, the rhinoviruses, has over a hundred members. Those viruses containing DNA are in the minority, and form the herpes family, the wart or papilloma viruses and the smallpox virus.

The RNA viruses are associated with such conditions as influenza, measles, mumps, rubella, diarrhoea, pneumonia, meningitis, hepatitis, polio and rabies. One group in particular, the *respiratory syncytial virus* or RSV, invades the respiratory tract of babies, who develop bronchitis and pneumonia at an early age, usually in the winter months of their first year and who may become severely ill. Another seasonal condition of babies is 'epidemic winter vomiting', in which there is vomiting and diarrhoea, often with dehydration, and in whom the wheel-shaped *rotavirus* appears in the stools. The *arboviruses* are so-called because they are transmitted by insects that live in the jungles (L. arbor = tree), particularly mosquitoes (yellow fever, dengue fever) and ticks (viral encephalitis). The *enteroviruses*, which live in the gut but exhibit symptoms elsewhere, include that of polio (the virus damages the nerve cells of the anterior horn of the lower spinal cord, thus paralysing the legs) and of the *Coxsackie virus* associated with hand foot and mouth disease (Coxsackie is a suburb of New York where the virus was first isolated).

The Herpes family

Of all the hundreds of viruses trying to make a living on the human race, none are more successful or enterprising than the herpes viruses (Gr. herpo = to creep). They have acquired the ability to hibernate for long periods inside a cell, sometimes for the whole of the host's lifetime, and break out when conditions are right to spread to others. Four groups of human herpes viruses are known: herpes simplex (cold sore), herpes varicella/zoster (chickenpox and shingles), Epstein-Barr virus (glandular fever) and the cytomegalovirus (CMV).

Herpes simplex is responsible for symptoms in a variety of different areas of the body but the basic lesion is always a blister. The initial attack, when the virus first establishes itself in the body, occurs either in the region of the face or the genitalia as a rule, and two slightly different strains of the virus are involved, herpes simplex I or HS1 *(herpes labialis)* in the mouth and HS2 or *herpes genitalis* on the genitals. The method of transmission is by contact, either oral for HS1 or sexual for HS2, and during the primary attack the symptoms are often so mild as to pass unnoticed. In some, however, the first attack is severe and there may be *stomatitis* with mouth ulcers, especially in young children. Occasionally the virus selects an unusual site, such as the cornea to cause a *dendritic ulcer* (see chapter 19), or the finger to cause a herpetic whitlow, or even a generalised infection of skin which is eczematous (eczema herpeticum).

Once the primary infection is over, the virus travels to a site on a nearby nerve ganglion where it remains in a dormant state until reactivated by a stimulus such as sunlight, cold or intercurrent illness. HS1 has a preference for the trigeminal ganglion, and when reactivated travels down the trigeminal nerve to a site on the face, usually the lips as they are more vulnerable. Here the virus irritates the cells to cause the familiar tingling sensation, followed by a blister which then crusts over and slowly heals. During the stage of blister-formation the virus can be passed to another person by direct contact, and in fact 19 people out of 20 actually carry the virus, although many are unaware of it.

HS2 is slightly different, in that it has a preference for the sacral nerve ganglion and produces identical ulcers on the penis, labia or cervix, which differ from those of syphilis by being painful and often multiple. In the event of cervical lesions, there will usually be a discharge and some generalised malaise and fever, and recurrent attacks damage the cells and predispose towards cervical cancer. Moreover, if a woman with active cervical herpes gives birth, there is a chance that the baby may develop a generalised herpes infection which is often fatal, and sometimes a Caesarian delivery will be recommended.

Herpes varicella/zoster (VZ) is the cause of both chickenpox and **shingles**. Chickenpox, described in more detail in the next section, is the primary infection of the virus and it is only when this reactivates that it produces the condition known as shingles, or herpes zoster. Once the child has recovered from chickenpox, the virus remains dormant in a cranial or spinal sensory root ganglion and many years later produces a blistering, painful rash over the area of distribution of the nerve, typically the ophthalmic division of the trigeminal nerve but sometimes affecting a small area of the trunk or abdomen where it forms a band around the body, 'a belt of roses from hell!'. If the attack is a severe one the blisters may later form deep scars and remain continually painful, *post-herpetic neuralgia*, and this is especially likely to occur in the elderly. Because the blisters of shingles contain the active virus, it is possible to contract the primary form of the disease – chickenpox – from a case, but not vice versa.

Glandular fever is a not uncommon condition found in teenagers and young adults. Labelled the 'kissing disease' by the popular press, it is indeed mostly passed on by salivary contact, but has a fairly long incubation period of about 4–6 weeks and does not cause epidemics but rather isolated cases. The cardinal symptoms are a fever, sore throat and swollen glands, so that initially it is very similar to acute tonsillitis with which it is easily confused. However, the course of glandular fever tends to be a protracted one, going on for months in many cases, with weakness, malaise, headaches and rather vague symptoms. Some distinguishing features of the disease are the appearance of swollen glands in other parts of the body, red spots on the palate, stiffness of the joints in some cases, and sometimes a rash on the body and puffiness around the eyes. In about half the cases there is enlargement of the liver or spleen, leading to mild hepatitis and even jaundice. In order to confirm the diagnosis blood is sent for examination of the lymphocytes which have abnormally large, misshapen nuclei (hence the alternative name for the disease of *infectious mononucleosis*) which are formed as a response to the presence of the *Epstein-Barr virus*, the source of the trouble. The EBVirus also stimulates the production of antibodies against it, and these can be detected by the monospot test.

Cytomegalovirus or CMV is an example of what is sometimes called 'opportunistic infection', that is it does not cause symptoms unless there is a considerable lowering of the resistance of the host. It is therefore most often seen in those patients who have had transplants and are immunosuppressed, or in those suffering from cancer or AIDS. They develop a condition similar to that of glandular fever, with hepatitis and even pneumonia. The name 'cytomegalovirus' derives from the enlarged cells seen in tissues infected with the organism.

Childhood Illness

During the months following birth a baby is protected from the majority of infectious diseases by the presence of maternal antibodies. By the age of about 6 months, however, these will have been lost by the natural process of degeneration and the infant will therefore be to some degree susceptible to infection. Once the infection has been contracted, the person will thereafter usually have lifelong immunity from that particular disease, although rarely they may get it twice.

Most childhood diseases are of viral origin, and spread through the community by droplet infection from coughing, or sometimes by actual contact (contagion). Only rarely are they contracted by water-borne or food-borne methods, except in the case of gastroenteritis which is discussed separately. Following the acquisition of the organism there is a period of a few days while it multiplies within the body to form sufficient numbers to cause symptoms, the *incubation period*. Towards the end of the incubation period, which differs in length according to the disease, there is a rise in temperature and general loss of well-being, before the onset of the symptoms specific to the disease itself, and this is known as the *prodromal period*.

Because the child is infectious during the prodromal period, and sometimes during the incubation period as well, the condition is quickly passed around the community, and small epidemics occur which if widespread and affecting other countries are known as 'pandemics'. Whether or not an epidemic happens depends largely on the level of immunity of the majority of the child population, and when this falls below about 50% then a new one is likely to break out, which happens every 4–5 years or so. In between some isolated cases occur but there are insufficient susceptible individuals around for the organism to establish itself.

Measles is associated with a virus and responsible for an enormous morbidity and mortality worldwide, especially where the host is in a poor state of health initially. It is responsible for 1% of total world deaths and is especially devastating in Africa. The virus affects chiefly the skin and respiratory tract, and is transmitted by droplet infection, having an incubation period of about 12 days. Children aged between 1 and 5 years are mostly involved, the first symptoms being non-specific fever and catarrh with a dry, croupy cough – the *catarrhal phase*. These are indistinguishable from a cold unless the mouth is examined, when the presence of *Koplik's spots* can be seen like small grains of sand on a deep red background opposite the molars on the mucus membrane of the cheek.

A day or two later the rash appears, the *exanthematous stage*, usually on the forehead and behind the ears as a pink, slightly raised series of small blotches. This spreads to the face and trunk, but rarely the limbs, and as it does so the spots become larger and confluent (joined together), lasting 4–7 days and then fading with slight scaling. There is accompanying *conjunctivitis* with watering and redness of the eyes which is mild but causes some photophobia (hence the old wives tale about light damaging the eyes). The main complication of measles is *otitis media* and the slight risk of perforation of the drum which seems to lead to chronic discharge in some. The mild *bronchitis* which is part of the disease may sometimes turn into a more severe chest infection with pneumonia, especially in the undernourished or immunosuppressed. Rarely, in about 1 in 1000 cases, there is progression to encephalitis after a week or so, and the patient becomes stuporose and convulsions may occur.

Fig. 3.1   *Koplik's spots*

Rubella or *German measles* is an altogether milder condition and although similar in some ways to measles is an unrelated virus. In about half the cases the rash does not appear or goes unnoticed as it is so brief, which is why many people have antibodies to the virus but are unaware of ever having had the disease. The remainder develop a mild prodromal phase with malaise and fever for a day or two, after incubating the virus for about 2–3 weeks, and then a faint, pink rash appears mostly on the trunk, but not as marked as the dusky blotches of measles. The rash lasts from a few hours to a few days, and there is often redness and watering of the eyes, and enlargement of the lymph nodes of the neck, especially those in the occipital area, and sometimes in other parts of the body too. In older girls and women there may be some stiffness of the joints which may persist for months, especially in the fingers or the knees, but this resolves without complication.

The main danger of rubella is when it occurs in mothers-to-be in the first three months of pregnancy when the cells of the foetus are differentiating to become the different organs and are very susceptible to the virus at this stage, particularly the heart and nervous system. This may result in congenital abnormalities such as heart lesions, deafness, cataract or mental handicap, especially if the infection was acquired within the first month of pregnancy (when the mother may even be unaware that she is pregnant). For this reason there is a policy to offer rubella immunisation to girls at the age of 12 or so.

Mumps is a glandular infection, again of viral aetiology, spread by droplet infection in the same way as measles and rubella. Here the incubation period is longer, about three weeks on average, followed usually by swelling of the salivary glands, most commonly one of the parotids but sometimes it may start in the submandibular. The gland is tender and swollen, and salivation may be uncomfortable so the pain is worse at mealtimes. If the inside of the mouth is inspected the red orifice of the parotid duct may be seen in a position very close to where Koplik's spots would be observed, beside the molars. Swelling of the salivary gland lasts a few days and then subsides, perhaps going to another or to the testes, ovaries or pancreas. Quite a number of children experience some abdominal pain from a mild degree of *pancreatitis*, and post-pubertal boys may experience inflammation of the testis (*orchitis*) in about 20% of cases, although only a very few, about 1%, develop sterility afterwards. A mild form of *meningitis* is sometimes seen as the glandular symptoms are resolving, when the child will complain of severe headache, drowsiness, neck stiffness and perhaps stupor. There may also be photophobia and vomiting, so any of these symptoms should alert one to the possibility. Fortunately the condition resolves without damage and most children make an uneventful recovery within a week or so.

Chickenpox or herpes varicella is a generalised febrile illness which may be caught by droplet infection or by contact with a blister of either another case of chickenpox or a case of shingles (which is the same virus appearing at a later stage). The incubation period is about two weeks, following which flat spots or *macules* appear on the trunk and sometimes the face and mouth but seldom much on the limbs. These soon progress to lumps or *papules* and then swell with clear fluid to form tiny blisters or *vesicles*. As these are very itchy they are generally scratched and become infected, so the clear fluid becomes pus (*pustules*) and finally scabs over and disappears, often leaving a scar crater, the whole process taking about a week. As well as the skin lesions the patient suffers from a general illness with headache, fever and limb pains, but these symptoms disappear as the crops of spots clear up, generally after about a week.

When chickenpox occurs in an adult it is usually of a more severe nature and the illness is more prolonged, with the risk of complications such as *varicella pneumonia* which develops within a few days of the eruption of spots, leading to a cough and sometimes haemoptysis. A form of *meningitis*, similar to that complicating mumps, may appear, but in this case is likely to be more severe and possibly leave permanent damage, particularly to the cerebellum causing ataxia (staggering). The complication of *shingles* has already been mentioned in the previous section.

Recently an indirect complication of chickenpox in particular has been described in children given aspirin for the fever. Known as *Reye's syndrome*, it is very uncommon but has a high mortality in the few who are afflicted by it, and may leave those who recover with a degree of brain damage. The drug causes damage to the liver and brain and produces symptoms of vomiting, drowsiness and eventually deep coma. Reye's syndrome is also seen in children with influenza and less often in other febrile illnesses, so it is now recommended that aspirin is never used by children with fevers.

Roseola is a mild and only slightly infectious illness of infants and young children, and a virus is suspected but has not been identified. The incubation is about 12 days and is followed by a mild fever and as this vanishes a faint, pink, macular rash appears on the neck and trunk lasting only a few hours. There are no complications to this common illness, and it is so similar in appearance to a mild case of rubella that the diagnosis is often unconfirmed.

Whooping cough is unlike most of the other childhood diseases in that it is probably caused by a bacterium, bordetella pertussis, rather than a virus and the symptoms continue for a considerable time, often amounting to several months. The condition is caught by droplet infection from someone in the catarrhal stage and this is followed by an incubation period of a week. The first evidence of illness is a runny nose and loose cough with slight fever, indistinguishable from a cold, but after a week or so this *catarrhal phase* changes to a *paroxysmal phase* as the mucus thickens and the infection descends into the lungs to plug the small bronchi. Great effort is required to expel the mucus and leads to the typical paroxysms of coughing followed by the inspiratory 'whoop' so typical of the disease. The spasm of coughing leads to cyanosis, salivation and often vomiting, occasionally with convulsions if there is sufficient lack of oxygen. Because of the very high pressure generated in the thorax by coughing, the eyes bulge and may haemorrhage or hernias may develop and even rectal prolapse. In between the attacks the child is able to breathe normally without coughing, and it is only in babies and young children that the disease is usually serious. Gradually the severity of the symptoms lessens, but a cough will often persist for months afterwards.

The complications of pertussis are uncommon but occasionally some sticky mucus will plug a bronchus completely so that the lung beyond it will collapse and a *lung abscess* form in the stagnant tissue, or a secondary *pneumonia* may occur. If the bronchi or their cilia become locally damaged, they tend to dilate and form small pockets of infection, a condition termed *bronchiectasis* (qv), leaving a continual disability. Serious neurological reactions, such as may follow pertussis immunisation, are very rare.

Scarlet fever is another illness where bacteria play a part, in this case a particular strain of *streptococcus* (see next section). This was once a greatly feared disease, running swiftly through communities and families and often rapidly fatal. Today it is a pale shadow of itself, possibly because the bacterium has undergone mutation, and the term *scarletina* is sometimes used instead. After an incubation period of 2–3 days the child develops a high temperature and a sore throat, often with enlarged tonsillar glands and infected tonsils. The next day a red rash like a flush starts behind the ears and spreads to involve the whole body, sparing the area around the mouth ('circumoral pallor'), as the muscle here is attached firmly to the skin. The redness is caused by a toxin secreted by the streptococcus. The tongue is initially furred, the 'white strawberry', but then peels to leave the typically 'red strawberry' tongue at the same time as the rash on the body fades and peels over a period of a week or so.

The two possible complications of scarlet fever are *rheumatic fever* and *acute nephritis*, both of which are rare but are described in the sections on heart and kidney disorders respectively.

Periods of Infectivity

For reference, the number of days for which a person should be regarded as infectious are as follows:

Measles: from onset of the catarrh until 4 days after the rash starts.
Rubella: from 7 days before the rash until 4 days after rash starts.
Mumps: from 7 days after the first swollen gland appears.
Chickenpox: from first symptoms until rash has started to scab.
Pertussis: from first catarrh until 3 weeks afterwards.
Scarlet fever: very variable, depending on duration of throat symptoms.

Bacteria and the Body

Bacteria, although larger than viruses, cannot really be classified in either the plant or animal kingdoms. They contain only a single chromosome in a primitive nucleus, and have a rigid cell wall which determines their shape. This shape is an important factor in classifying bacteria, and takes the form of spheres (*cocci*), rods (*bacilli*) or spirals (*spirochaetes*). Unlike viruses, many bacteria are able to survive for long periods in adverse conditions by hibernating as spores, rather like the seeds of a plant.

The cocci, when examined microscopically, like to group themselves into either clusters if they are *staphylococci* (Gr. staphys = bunch of grapes), in rows if they are *streptococci* (Gr. streptos = chain) or in pairs if they are *diplococci*, such as the gonococcus and the meningococcus.

Staphylococci are the great pus-forming organisms, pus being the debris of phagocytes and dead bacteria, and they are therefore seen in *boils, abscesses, styes, wound infections, impetigo* and many other conditions, including *food poisoning*. There are many different members of the family, some quite innocent which live on the skin, and some potentially pathogenic (harmful), often living in the nose. It is from here that they may be shed to cause skin infections and boils in the susceptible (which is why masks are worn in hospitals), and many are resistant to some antibiotics such as penicillin from whose clutches they escape by producing an enzyme, B lactamase, which destroys it. Occasionally staphylococci gain entry from a skin infection into the blood, and a septicaemia or blood-poisoning occur with the possibility of metastatic abscesses forming in other parts of the body, such as the joints, lungs or bones.

A condition known as the *toxic shock syndrome* is thought to arise from the invasion of staphs through the vaginal wall which has been damaged or dehydrated through the use of modern super-absorbent tampons, and which leads to sudden collapse with vomiting, fever and a rash at the time of menstruation.

Streptococci produce large numbers of different toxins, enzymes which destroy the body's defences in some manner, either by breaking down the cement which holds the cells together, enabling the bacterium to spread rapidly under the skin (as in cellulitis and erysipelas), or by producing an 'erythrogenic toxin' which causes the red rash of scarlet fever and the 'strep throat'. Many streptococci are able to break up or 'haemolyse' the red blood cells, and this is used as the basis of their classification into different groups named the Lancefield groups. Streptococci are involved in such various conditions as *tonsillitis and sore throats, scarlet fever, otitis media, lobar pneumonia* (in the form of the pneumococcus) and *puerperal fever*. They appear to have moderated their behaviour towards humans in the last few decades, however, in that they are by no means as virulent probably because of mutation. They are also very susceptible to penicillin and do not produce resistant strains. Following an infection with one particular streptococcus, the Lancefield group A variety, an individual may subsequently develop one of three separate conditions due to the production of antibodies which unfortunately act against the body's own tissues. These tissues are the heart, particularly the heart valves, to cause *rheumatic fever*, the glomerulus of the kidney to cause *nephritis*, and the skin of the legs to cause the characteristic blotchy rash of *erythema nodosum*.

The diplococcus is a bean-shaped bacterium which tends to exist in pairs, perhaps because as the *gonococcus* it is associated with gonorrhoea and can be seen in the urethral or vaginal discharge of cases of this disease. A slightly different diplococcus, the *meningococcus*, is seen in the CSF of cases of bacterial meningitis. Recently both have developed a degree of resistance to many antibiotics.

The Bacilli. There are numerous very different rod-shaped members of this genus a few of which, like the tetanus and gangrene organisms, are able to survive anaerobically without the need for oxygen and live in the soil and decaying matter. These are members of the family *clostridium*, some of which, notably the botulism bacillus, produce the most powerful poisons known. It has been estimated that enough botulinum toxin to kill the population of the UK could be contained on the head of a pin, making it probably the most lethal substance in existence.

Most bacilli, however, require oxygen to survive, such as the mycobacterium family which are known as *acid-fast bacilli* because of their ability to resist strong acids, and which comprise the leprosy and tuberculosis organisms. A much larger family is that of the enterobacteria or *coliforms* because they live in the gut. They include bacillary dysentery, typhoid, plague and of course the well-known E.coli which causes problems especially if it strays into the urinary tract. Other bacilli are the comma-shaped vibrio of cholera, the whooping cough bacillus and brucellosis.

Spirochaetes. These spiral bacteria are best known for their relationship with *syphilis* and *yaws* (a tropical disease very similar to syphilis), and these types are known as Treponema. Another type of spirochaete, Leptospira, is seen in a severe form of jaundice found in canal and sewage workers – *Weil's disease* or *leptospirosis*.

Chlamydia. As well as the three main groups of bacteria, there are several groups of rather smaller organisms which fall midway in size between bacteria and viruses. One of the better known of these is the chlamydia, a furry little beast named after the Latin 'chlamys' meaning a hair shirt, and thought to be involved in the

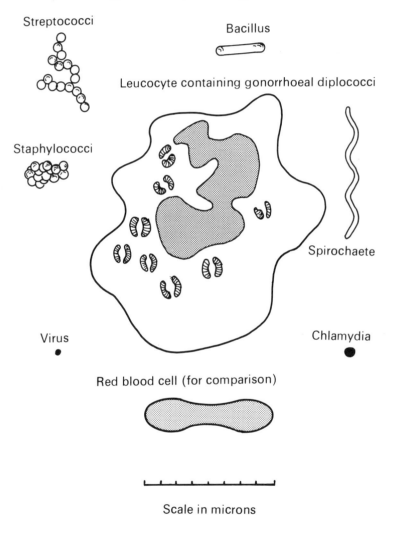

Fig. 3.2   *The relative size of some organisms*

condition known as *non-specific urethritis* or NSU, the commonest form of sexually transmitted disease. The very same
organism also features in certain eye conditions under the name
of 'inclusion conjunctivitis' seen in children after they have been
swimming, or in adults who may acquire it indirectly from the
genital tract. The eye disease *trachoma* is probably its most
notorious manifestation world-wide, and is a common cause of
blindness in Third World countries (see chapter 19).

Another form of chlamydia occurs in the form of *psittacosis*,
one of the so-called 'atypical pneumonias' and seen in those who
handle certain birds, particularly parrots, budgerigars and ducks.

Diarrhoea and Gastroenteritis

The digestive tract, like the respiratory tract, is constantly in
contact with the environment and is thus liable to contamination
by allergy, poisoning and infection. The reaction of the body is
to attempt to rid itself of the offending food, which it does by
vomiting and diarrhoea, common symptoms of all types of 'food
poisoning'. Infections are seen much more in countries where
hygiene and water-supplies are inadequate, often resulting from
parasites such as amoebas and giardias which may remain in the
gut, whereas the consumption of chemicals and antibiotics are
the main cause of such symptoms in the West. Nor is it usually
possible to distinguish chemical from infective causes from the
nature of the symptoms alone, and consideration of the diet is
necessary. However, as treatment is largely a question of
replacement of the fluid lost with dilute fruit juice (but no sugar),
the distinction is mostly irrelevant.

Diarrhoea in Babies and Infants.

In young babies gastroenteritis may lead to dehydration if severe,
when they are initially irritable, pale and thirsty but only passing
a small volume of urine. Later the skin loses its elasticity and the
tongue becomes dry, with sunken eyes and fontanelles. By this
time the child is quite severely ill, and may become cyanosed and
collapse, so intravenous fluid may be needed if the baby
continues to vomit. Breast feeding gives considerable protection
against infections as the baby absorbs antibodies from the
mother, as well as having a perfectly balanced diet.

Severe attacks of gastroenteritis occasionally occur in neonatal wards, caused by a pathogenic strain of E. coli, the normal gut commensal, which is spread rapidly during nursing procedures and carries a high mortality. Babies and infants are also liable to rotavirus infection which occurs in sporadic outbreaks as *epidemic winter vomiting,* often accompanied by a cough and a cold as the virus also inflames the respiratory tract. Even after the acute illness has been overcome the cells of the small intestine are left damaged and unable to produce the enzyme lactase needed to digest milk, so when this is reintroduced into the feed the stools remain loose and frothy. Milk should therefore be avoided for 2–3 weeks after severe diarrhoea until the *lactase deficiency* has been restored.

Sometimes other infections such as *otitis media, pneumonia or meningitis* may present as diarrhoea or vomiting, and evidence of these conditions should be looked for.

Diarrhoea in Children and Adults.

In this age group diarrhoea is often mild and due to an inappropriate diet or sometimes an enterovirus ('gastric flu'). Certain foods such as undercooked red beans, poisonous fungi, shellfish and mackerel contain potential poisons which may give rise to symptoms. Food which has begun to decompose will form amines called ptomaines, and before the advent of refrigerators this was an occasional source of food poisoning.

Staphylococcal food poisoning may follow the consumption of food contaminated with these organisms, which are present on the skin of an infected food-handler and which contain a tasteless toxin which is resistant to heat, so that the toxin may still exist even though the bacteria have been killed. It is this type of food poisoning which leads to the sudden severe stomach cramps experienced by aircraft passengers, for instance, when a whole batch of food becomes contaminated by the organism. The symptoms, though dramatic, seldom last more than 24–48 hours, and there is no accompanying fever. A similar toxin-mediated condition is caused by *bacillus cereus*, a bacterium which has a preference for cooked rice and is sometimes an unwelcome extra in a take-away meal.

Consuming infected meat or milk may result in a condition named *campylobacter enteritis* after the organism involved. Outbreaks occur particularly in schools or are contracted from pets, and are characterised by a slow onset of fever, nausea, muscular pains and abdominal pain, sometimes confused with appendicitis. This is followed by profuse, often bloodstained, diarrhoea the next day which may be so severe as to cause incontinence.

Salmonella gastroenteritis is another condition seen after consumption of infected food, especially meat and poultry, and is becoming increasingly common. The usual way of contracting it is through frozen produce which has not been thoroughly heated while cooking. Symptoms are diarrhoea, usually with vomiting, fever and colicky abdominal pain, and sometimes severe illness with shock and dehydration in the elderly. About 5% of sufferers continue to harbour the organism in the gallbladder after they have recovered, and excrete it in the stools as carriers.

Diarrhoea in Travellers.

Those who travel to certain parts of the world are at increased risk of infection from organisms in the locality, as well as from the alteration of their diet which may in itself cause symptoms. So-called *traveller's diarrhoea* (Delhi belly, Montezuma's revenge) is a result of contact with a strain of E. coli with which the gut is unfamiliar but which is local to the area and therefore does not cause symtoms to the indigenous population. The diarrhoea is sudden, usually mild and self-limiting after a few days once the intestine has become colonised. Although often labelled 'dysentery', this name should really be reserved for a different disease related to the bacillus Shigella (*bacillary dysentery*). The shigella species come in different types, some of which are quite virulent and cause the life-threatening bloody diarrhoea of the tropics such as Kipling describes so vividly, while others are involved in a relatively mild disorder.

Cholera was once a relatively common European disease despite being known as the 'Asiatic cholera', but is now only seen in certain areas of the world, mostly the Ganges basin. The comma-shaped vibrio periodically mutates and spreads in world-wide pandemics, of which we are now in the seventh, El Tor, variety. Spread is through the contamination of drinking water by sewage as a rule, and when this is drunk then a few days later there may be abdominal pain and severe watery diarrhoea in enormous volume ('rice water stools'), so most deaths come from the inevitable dehydration. The reason for this is that the vibrio secretes a toxin which prevents the intestinal cells from absorbing any salt or water, thereby losing it from the body.

Typhoid and *paratyphoid*, collectively known as the *enteric fevers*, are not primarily diarrhoeal disorders but it is convenient to discuss them here. Both are due to varieties of salmonella, but the illness is generally much more severe and prolonged. Like salmonella, it can be contracted from carriers directly but more often is a result of consuming infected food or water. The bacteria can survive gastric acid and then penetrate the wall of the intestine to get into the lymphatics from where they are spread all over the body in the blood stream. This results in the typical symptoms of fever with rigors, headache and a dry cough, often with abdominal pains also, and then as the illness progresses the rose-coloured spots appear on the skin and the spleen becomes enlarged. It is after this that the diarrhoea starts, by which time the patient is extremely ill with weakness and mental confusion, and there is a risk of the bowel perforating and causing peritonitis.

Two forms of diarrhoea found commonly in tropical countries are caused by protozoa which exist freely in both food and water, and to which the local population are to some extent immune. *Amoebic dysentery* starts as a diarrhoea with colicky pains and abdominal distension, and may become chronic despite treatment in the susceptible, when the diarrhoea continues or may become chronic constipation. The amoebas are liable to travel in the portal system to the liver and there form multiple abscesses ('amoebic hepatitis'), but this is not a common complication. They may also cause permanent damage to the gut wall which becomes stripped of its villi with the result that malabsorption occurs, a condition which is still sometimes known as 'tropical sprue'. *Giardiasis* is another protozoal condition, caused by Giardia lamblia, which also occurs in temperate countries such as Britain and the USA where it contaminates water and leads to outbreaks of abdominal pain, distension after food and diarrhoea. In children it may become chronic and destroy the villi of the small intestine to cause malabsorption (see chapter 13).

Infestations

As well as the micro-organisms there are two groups of animals which may infest the skin and intestines of man – the insects and worms respectively. Although often irritating and sometimes debilitating, they seldom cause serious disease but may be difficult to eradicate as the immune system is unable to make antibodies against them.

The *scabies mite* is spread by close, often sexual, contact between people, and burrows under the skin to cause intense itching, particularly at night when the warmth encourages the mites to move about. The lesions tend to start in between the fingers and on the wrists, sometimes in the groin area. Later they travel to other parts of the body and no part is exempt. On close inspection the tiny burrows made by the mite can be seen, terminating in a blister, although if scratching is severe these become obliterated and infected, sometimes leading to *impetigo* (qv). As well as using an insecticide to destroy the mites, the clothes and bedding must also be well washed to prevent reinfection.

Lice are another form of insect parasite but live only on the hairy parts of the body, different varieties being closely adapted to certain areas and races, even to the extent of having specially shaped claws to cling to the hair of different races. Pubic lice or *crabs* are found in the pubic hair and, like scabies, are spread mostly by sexual contact. They may also travel to other parts of the body such as the axillae or even eyebrows but not the hair on the head which is the province of head lice, usually seen in schoolchildren. The eggs of the head louse are found around the nape of the neck as small grey *nits* attached to the hair about halfway along, and these take about two weeks to hatch so the treatment must be repeated after a fortnight as only the lice are killed.

Threadworms are also mainly seen in children who ingest the eggs in contaminated soil, often through chewing their finger-nails. The eggs hatch in the intestine after two weeks or so, and the worm emerges from the anus at night to lay eggs on the skin, causing irritation of the area as it does so. The scratching causes contamination of the fingers and if these are not washed the whole cycle starts again.

4

Skin: Disorders of Protection

Our skin is much more than just an impervious envelope enclosing the body, it is a complete organ in itself. Its functions include controlling body temperature, sensing the world around, screening the sun's rays with the pigment melanin, insulating the body with a layer of fat, manufacturing vitamin D, secreting certain unwanted substances and signalling our emotional states by flushing whether we like it or not. There are even areas of specialised skin – the hair and nails – for different protective functions, and one or more of these may malfunction in a variety of ways. Skin disorders are numerous and many reflect abnormalities of the internal workings of the body, but they can be categorised according to the underlying contribution they make and the tissues affected.

The Eczemas

The term eczema literally means 'to boil over', and well describes the irritation and redness that takes place in the various forms of this condition, of which there are several types.

Atopic eczema is perhaps the best known, being a largely inherited predisposition to such allergic states as asthma and hay fever. It is thought that there is a transient deficiency of the local immunoglobulins in the gut mucosa during the first few months of life, which is when atopic eczema often starts, and that this allows food allergens to enter the blood and cause widespread stimulation of other antibodies which are situated in the epidermis. This partly explains the low incidence in breast-fed babies. Atopic eczema is usually worst in the skin creases of the elbows, knees and wrists (which is why it is sometimes known as *flexural eczema*), but it is also seen on the face, neck and trunk. By the age of 10, about 90% of children will have cleared up apart from the most severe cases. If the eczema is scratched it may become infected and develop *secondary impetigo*, and if an eczematous child contracts a cold sore he or she is liable to have a widespread and dangerous eruption wherever there is eczema (*eczema herpeticum*).

If a particular area of skin is scratched incessantly it will become thickened and rough, and is then described as having become *lichenified*, a term used for a number of disorders where the epidermis comes to resemble lichen. *Lichen simplex* or neurodermatitis is such a type of thickened eczema localised to one area of skin which is abraded incessantly either through habit (e.g. the neck or wrist), or because of sweating (pruritus ani & vulvae) or even localised atopic eczema. It is seen especially in overstressed individuals as a well-defined ridge of purple skin.

A similar situation occurs in *varicose eczema* where the underlying irritant is blood leaking from dilated varicose veins around the ankles, which discolours the skin a dull slate-grey and dries it up, leading eventually to cracking and ulceration.

Pompholyx eczema (Gr. pomphos = bubble) occurs mainly in young adults, especially those whose hands and feet sweat. It generally starts on the sides of the fingers as small, itchy, symmetrical blisters and may spread to the palms or soles before drying out and cracking to form chronic fissures. In most cases it is due to exposure to chemicals and detergents during housework etc, but in some is a reaction to fungal infections of the feet or to the ingestion of excess nickel found in some stainless steel pans.

Not all inflammations of the skin are eczemas, occasionally large blisters appear on the epidermis and in the mouth for no determinable reason and rupture to leave painful raw areas – *pemphigus*. Another inflammatory condition, more itchy than painful, is *lichen planus*. As the name suggests the lesions are raised and irregular, being a shiny pink or purple colour and found mostly on the wrists, shins and sacrum. They last for several months and then resolve, and are accompanied by a painless rash in the mouth consisting of a white, lacework pattern of spots and streaks which are of great help in diagnosing the rash.

Dermatitis and Urticaria

The skin responds to stimulation from chemicals, trauma,

temperature change and some foods in a variety of ways, the chief of which are by becoming inflamed (dermatitis) or swelling up (urticaria). The terms 'eczema' and 'dermatitis' are often used interchangeably, but technically the word 'dermatitis' means the type of eczema which follows directly or indirectly from contact with a chemical substance, while 'eczema' should be reserved for the constitutional types described in the last section.

Dermatitis is the inevitable consequence of contamination of the skin by certain substances, such as bleach, cement, washing powders, certain oils and dyes, and a rash will appear within a short time if protection is not used. Nappy rash caused by the ammonia in urine is an example. Other substances lead to allergies which do not manifest immediately but appear as dermatitis a week or so later. What happens is that following contact with the substance a small amount penetrates the skin and is passed to the local lymph nodes where antibodies are formed a few days later. The antibody then makes its way back to the epidermis and reacts with any remaining allergen it finds there to cause an area of irritation. In some cases the rash is more generalised and affects mostly the thinner skin of the eyelids, backs of the hands and fronts of the elbows to give puffiness and erythema (redness). When this happens the allergen may have long gone and be untraceable, but is commonly topical antibiotics or other creams, lanolin, rubber, chrome, nickel or plants such as primulas and poison ivy.

A special case, *photodermatitis*, is where the sensitised skin only reacts to the drug or other chemical where it is exposed to the sun, so the rash is restricted usually to the backs of the hands and the face. It seems that these substances enable sunburn to occur with even a small dose of UV light.

Urticaria is an itchy, blotchy, transient rash characterised by swelling of the skin or mucus membrane involved. This is brought about by an increase in the permeability of the vessels after histamine has been liberated in their vicinity, either by damage to the mast cells by allergens (similar to asthma) or by direct injection. Some types of food such as shellfish, straw-berries, nuts, fish and a host of food additives may lead a few minutes or hours later to a general reaction in the skin which comes out in wheals very similar to those caused by nettles but larger. Because the dermis rather than the epidermis is involved, the swelling is pronounced compared to dermatitis, and may reach very large proportions if the tissues of the lip, tongue, face, throat or eyelids are involved when the condition is sometimes referred to as *angio-oedema*.

Some, who are very susceptible, may go on to chronic urticaria when they are seldom free of the rash which comes on in response to physical stimuli such as cold, sunburn or pressure. There is likely to be sensitivity to certain foods and an exclusion diet may be needed to discover what can be tolerated. Not uncommonly they exhibit the symptom of *dermographism*, when stroking the skin will evoke a typical weal and flare response.

One specific type of urticaria, *papular urticaria*, also known as *heat bumps*, is that caused by the bites of insects, particularly fleas. The rash takes the form of recurrent eruptions of itchy papules all over the trunk which fade within a few days only to reappear infuriatingly after the next bite. The body has become allergic to the saliva of the flea, and usually it is the family pet that gets the blame although fleas commonly lurk in old furniture and carpets.

Disorders of Keratinisation — Psoriasis

Normally the epidermal cells are continually being formed in the deepest layers and migrating outwards to be shed at the surface. As they develop they are becoming hardened by a protein called keratin which also causes the cells to die, and in places subject to continual wear such as the palms and soles and wherever *calluses* form, the keratin layer builds up a greater thickness for protection. If such a callus develops at a point of pressure on the toe it may press on the nerve below to cause pain and is known as a *corn*.

Psoriasis is a mysterious condition of unknown cause whereby the rate of keratinisation of the epidermal cells is greatly speeded up, so that instead of taking a month to reach the surface they accomplish it in a few days and in doing so the process of keratinisation is inadequate, and so the cells all stick together. The result is that the thickened skin has a silvery, scaly appearance and flakes off prematurely to leave a pink, patchy, map-like rash underneath. This may be very disfiguring but, despite the name (psora means 'to itch'), not usually especially itchy. The condition affects about 2% of the population to some extent, but rarely starts before the teens and usually improves with age. Sometimes emotional or physical trauma or infectious disease is the precipitating factor, and there may be a family history.

Favoured sites are the prominences of the elbows and knees, the sacrum and the scalp especially at the hair line around the edge, but nowhere is immune. It is often symmetrical on the left and right sides of the body, and may arise at the site of trauma or an operation scar, (the *Koebner phenomenon*). Because of the different manner of keratinisation of the palms and soles, psoriasis is uncommon here but in those in whom it does occur it resembles large sterile pustules, *pustular psoriasis.* One common complication in about half of the cases is damage to the nails, usually as small craters in the surface called *pitting*, sometimes as separation of the nail bed or distortion. About one in fifteen sufferers develop an arthritis in one or more joints, often involving the fingers – *psoriatic arthritis.*

Ichthyosis is an uncommon condition seen mainly in cold, dry climates in young children, in most of whom it is inherited. The skin takes on a dry, scaly, fish-like appearance (Gr. ichtheus = fish) which in some cases is associated with the condition of atopic eczema and causes itching of especially the face and upper arms where it is prominent. Attention should be given to the diet which may be deficient in nicotinamide. A similar condition called *tylosis* affects only the palms and soles which are greatly thickened ('hyperkeratosis').

Sebaceous Disorders – Acne

The sebaceous glands secrete a greasy substance, sebum, on to the hairs of both body and scalp for protection not only against water but also to discourage fungal infections such as ringworm (which is why it is children who generally get scalp ringworm as their glands are less developed). The rate of secretion of sebum depends largely on stimulation from the sex hormones, especially androgens. Oestrogens tend to lessen the flow, which is why women often notice a fluctuation during their menstrual cycle, but the small amount of testosterone which they produce is sufficient to stimulate the glands.

Acne is one of the main consequences of seborrhoea (literally the flow of sebum), and occurs because the glands do not operate by secretion, but rather by allowing the cells of the lining to coagulate into a mass and form the sebum. The narrow opening through the hair follicle becomes blocked by debris, and this gradually changes colour until it is the familiar *blackhead* or *comedo*. The latter name derives from the assumption by the ancients that these were some kind of maggot which was eating into the flesh, and means 'a glutton'. If the problem is limited to these comedones then a few minutes in front of a mirror will do the trick, but unfortunately the accumulated sebum is an ideal medium for certain strains of bacilli which exist on the skin, and these multiply within the sebaceous gland to cause the familiar pustules or 'whiteheads' on the face, back and chest. In the most severe forms of acne the inflammation extends through the walls of the glands into the subcutaneous tissues to form pus-filled cysts which may coalesce, leading to severe scarring called *cystic acne*. Even young babies are not immune and their developing sebaceous glands may incur quite marked spottiness termed *infantile acne* which does, however, remit spontaneously after a few months.

Rosacea is a somewhat similar condition and at one time went by the name of *acne rosacea*, although it is doubtful now that the problem lies in the sebaceous gland, indeed no-one seems to be quite sure where it does lie. Nevertheless, the appearances are broadly similar with red pustules forming on the cheeks and around the mouth especially, sometimes moving to the forehead or nose. The skin takes on a flushed, mottled look with dilated, broken vessels and the peculiar fleshy swelling of the nose known as *rhinophyma*, seen only in men and usually ascribed quite erroneously to intemperance. A complication of this condition, seen mostly in women, is chronic conjunctivitis and persistant redness of the eyes.

Seborrhoeic eczema is a term used to describe a type of red, scaly and somewhat greasy rash common in babies and the elderly and largely restricted to the scalp (where it forms a severe type of *dandruff*) or the body folds (where it is termed *intertrigo*). Again there is no evidence that sebum secretion plays a part in the aetiology of the condition, but the distribution on the scalp and the body folds might lead one to suspect this. It particularly affects babies in whom it is seen around the eyes as *blepharitis*, behind the ears, in the groins as a severe form of *nappy rash*, and on the scalp as *cradle cap*. Quite often it becomes infected with yeasts such as Candida, and the tell-tale sign is when small 'satellite lesions' appear at the periphery of the rash.

Viral Infections – Warts

The epidermis reacts to many viruses by producing excrescences of tissue in the form of warts. Most of these viruses fall into the category of human papilloma viruses (HPV), the name papilloma being used for any kind of benign tumour of the skin. Nor does HPV only involve the skin, for it is found also on the mucus membranes of the genitals as genital or venereal warts.

The common wart seen on the fingers is a curious subject, apparently plagueing some individuals for months while leaving others untouched, sometimes emerging at the site of an injury (the Koebner phenomenon again), and sometimes taking the very smooth appearance of a planar wart on the face. When situated on the sole of the foot it is termed a *verruca* or plantar wart and sometimes covers large areas with hard, thickened skin (*mosaic wart*), and is often painful as the pressure drives it deep into the dermis.

A different strain of virus is seen in the penile and vulval warts known as *condylomata acuminata* (literally 'pointed knuckles') because of their irregular cauliflower-like shapes. These are almost always spread by sexual contact and often appear at the same time as other venereal conditions; they are also a factor in the aetiology of cervical cancer.

Children in particular are liable to crops of pearly-grey, firm swellings on the face or trunk. These are *molluscum contagiosum*, a type of wart in which a much larger virus may be found and which contains thick, cheesy material which can be expressed through the tiny dimple which surmounts the top. These warts are usually 2-10 in number and are about the size of a split pea.

Pityriasis rosea is the rather fanciful name given to a disorder which is thought to be due to a virus, and which often occurs in children. The word comes from the Greek meaning 'bran-like' and describes the speckled appearance of the fully-fledged rash. The first indication that something is happening is the appearance on the trunk of a pink, oval patch known as the *herald patch*, as it precedes the rash proper by several days. The child is usually perfectly well in himself and is often thought to have ringworm until the typical macular speckles appear on the trunk like an inverted Christmas tree, following the lines of the ribs. These last several weeks but eventually disappear leaving no ill-effects, nor is the child apparently infectious as the cases are invariably isolated ones.

Bacterial Infections – Impetigo

Large numbers of bacteria and yeasts populate the skin but seldom cause trouble unless there is underlying damage caused by sweating, scratching etc., when unwanted streptococci and staphylococci may arrive.

Impetigo is one of the more common consequences of either of these organisms and leads to a spreading infection of the epidermis when serum oozes from the raw surface and congeals as the typical honey-coloured crusts, moving about from one part of the body to another in a highly contagious fashion but seen especially around the mouth of children.

Some types of streptococci contain toxins which enable them to break down the connective tissue and spread rapidly across the skin as may happen in the *cellulitis* which follows some insect bites, and is extremely painful. When this happens to the tissues of the face this is termed *erysipelas* and leads to much oedema and swelling as the skin here is very loose and thin.

Staphylococci on the skin may inflame particularly the tiny glands attached to the hairs which secrete grease, and these then swell with pus. If this happens generally on the beard area it is called *barber's rash* or *sycosis barbae* as it is spread by shaving. Other parts of the body where hairs are found are liable to infection as *boils* or *styes*, and if the hair is removed they will discharge pus. If the boil is so large that it has several discharging orifices then it is called a *carbuncle*, and these kind of infections are particularly likely to occur in diabetics. Recurrent crops of boils (*furunculosis*) may result from malnutrition or poor diet, since the bacteria are able to reside symptomlessly in the nose and be spread by sneezing.

Fungal Infections – Ringworm

Fungi are the most frequent unwelcome guests on our skin, usually those from the ringworm (Tinea) family. There are four main species involved with humans, and they seem to have their own preferred areas of activity.

Tinea pedis or *athletes foot* is pretty much restricted to the spaces between the toes in those who sweat profusely or are careless about drying themselves after a shower. The fungus is readily found on the floors of changing rooms etc. and in a few people will provoke a more general type of allergic reaction – the 'id' reaction – and cause irritation of other parts of the skin, including pompholyx.

Tinea corporis is seen on the trunk or limbs as a pink, raised area which gradually expands over a few days, clearing in the centre as it does so. This gives it the appearance of a ring similar to that formed by the 'fairy ring' of toadstools, and it is from this that the name *ringworm* derives (it was once thought to be an actual worm). In time satellite lesions appear around the edge, which helps to distinguish it from eczema, and the rash becomes itchy and is readily spread among schoolchildren. A very similar type of ringworm, *Tinea capitis*, can be caught from animals like dogs and cats and affects mainly the scalp. An inflamed and itchy area develops and the hair may be lost in a manner similar to alopecia from which it must be differentiated.

Lastly comes *Tinea cruris* or *dhobi itch*, which affects the area around the groin and armpits, and is caught in a manner similar to that of athletes foot, especially in the tropics. The name derives from the custom of Indian dhobis to wash the clothes in the nearest pond, and then starch them well which provided an excellent medium for the fungi and some embarrassing moments for the Raj!

A fungus distantly related to Tinea may affect the skin of those who holiday in the sun and come back with an unusual tan. It is discussed in the next section under pigmentation disorders.

Disorders of Pigmentation – *Vitiligo*

The colour of the skin is determined by the presence of the pigment melanin formed in the melanocytes of the basal layer of the epidermis. This dark brown pigment is extruded into the epidermal cells where it protects the sensitive nuclei of the epidermal cells from damage and possible malignant change from the ultraviolet radiation emitted by the sun. It is packed together more densely in those races who come from hot climates and who thus have a darker skin. The enzymes which produce melanin are activated by UV light, so exposure does tan the skin but as the epidermis is shed over the following weeks this tan goes with it. Nor is the current trend of exposing oneself more fully and more frequently to the elements without a certain risk of malignant change in later life, especially in the case of fair-skinned people in whom the melanin is distributed somewhat unevenly as collections of melanocytes better known as *freckles*.

Vitiligo is the patchy loss of pigmentation which is most obvious in coloured people to whom it may be a source of great embarrassment, not least because it superficially resembles the depigmentation seen in leprosy. The word comes from the Latin 'vitellus' meaning a calf and was used by the Roman physician Celsus to describe the resemblance to the white spots on a calf's legs. The melanocytes in certain areas atrophy and even die leaving a widespread, symmetrical pattern all over the body. The condition is quite common, affecting about 1 person in 50 to some degree, and appears to be increasing. It is more common in those with autoimmune disorders such as pernicious anaemia and thyroid disease, and antibodies against melanocytes have been demonstrated.

A similar loss of pigment occurs for a completely different reason in *pityriasis versicolour*, and the two conditions are sometimes confused. However this variety of pityriasis is a fungal problem, arising on the neck and trunk of those who holiday in the sun, and leads to an unexpected mottling of their tan until it fades. The acid produced by the fungus bleaches the melanin in small, localised areas and it tends to recur each year in the susceptible.

Hair and Nail Disorders – Alopecia

Hairs consist of tubes of keratin which sprout from very active hair papillae at the roots where the cells are dividing at an enormous rate. This rate of growth is by no means always constant, however, and after growing to a length of 2–3 feet, which may take several years, the hair is shed and replaced by a new one. All this happens in a random pattern so that every day up to 100 hairs are lost from the head. In animals there is a more cyclical shedding which takes the form of moulting, but in humans this only happens after a severe illness, emotional trauma or pregnancy when there is a sudden thinning of the hair a few weeks later, followed by renewal.

Alopecia is the name given to patchy hair loss with well-defined edges (Gr. alopix = a mangy fox), and is seen on the scalp or beard area. It frequently starts in childhood but may occur at any age and the patches may be single or multiple and are usually about the size of a 50p piece. After a few months the hair generally starts to grow again but is often a lighter shade for a while. A few people develop alopecia of the whole scalp or even the whole body, in which case recovery is unlikely. Around the edge of the bald area are short stumpy hairs with a swollen base – *exclamation mark hairs!* – which enable this condition to be distinguished from other causes such as ringworm of the scalp, hair pulling etc.

The cause of alopecia is thought to be an auto-immune process affecting the hair follicles and in some cases there is an association with vitiligo. It is also more common in those who have Down's syndrome.

Like the hair, the nails are also outgrowths of keratin, and like hair they also develop air spaces in them which turns them white, and this is seen especially in those who are short of the mineral zinc. The nail bed, which is just behind the cuticle, is where the nails form so any trauma here is likely to leave a legacy for some three months while the nail grows out. It is seen as either a midline groove in those who pick their cuticle, or as a transverse line (Beau's line) in those whose nails temporarily stop growing during a severe illness. More severe damage results in the nail becoming greatly thickened and curved, seen especially in the toes of jockeys and stable lads.

Discolouration of the nail is common, especially in those who enjoy gardening, when strands of fungi may become lodged in the cracks and gradually turn the nail yellow, green or brown, pervading the keratin and separating it from its bed. A similar fungal disorder affects those who immerse their hands in water frequently and causes inflammation of the cuticle (*paronychia*) which becomes red and soggy. In cases of liver and kidney

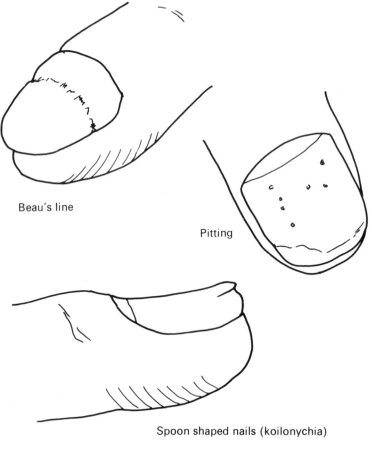

Beau's line

Pitting

Spoon shaped nails (koilonychia)

Fig. 4.1   *Examples of nail pathology*

disease, where there is a reduction in the serum proteins, the nail may become very pale or even quite white, and sometimes this is confined to the half moons at the proximal aspect of the nail.

Distortion of the nail is seen particularly in severe iron deficiency when there is a *spoon-shaped*, dry, brittle nail which cracks easily ('koilonychia'), and this also occurs in myxoedema. Psoriasis leads to the familiar pitting of nails by involving the nail bed, and sometimes even lifts the nail off its bed altogether and discolours it.

Skin Tumours

Lumps appearing on the skin may arise from one or more of a number of structures and this has given rise to a variety of descriptive terms such as 'naevus', 'mole', 'wart', etc which are not always accurate and do not always distinguish between benign and malignant lesions.

Benign Tumours

At birth almost all babies have some form of skin blemish ranging from the common 'stork mark' of dilated capillaries on the neck or the bridge of the nose, to the *'strawberry mark'* or cavernous naevus which is sometimes quite large but almost always disappears by the fifth year of life. Occasionally babies are born with an extensive capillary naevus with a network of dilated capillaries called the *port wine stain* which persists. Incidentally the word 'naevus' actually means 'mole' in Latin but has come to refer to tumours involving the vessels.

Moles are collections of melanocytes, the pigment-containing cells of the skin, which usually develop in the course of a lifetime, sometimes in large numbers. If one is present at birth then it tends to cause distortion of the hair follicles in that area resulting in a tuft of coarse hair surmounting it. Moles take many shapes and sizes and are often multiple, ranging from light pink to dark brown. Only very rarely do they become malignant (see below) and this is more likely where they are large or deeply pigmented. In old age a rather peculiar type of benign but very warty-looking mole may develop, particularly on the temples, neck or trunk. These are known as *seborrheic* or *senile warts* and have a greasy apppearance, sometimes reaching an inch or more in diameter.

Sebaceous cysts, or 'wens' as they are sometimes called, are cysts of the sebaceous glands attached to the hair follicles and are thus found principally on the scalp where they grow to look like a round grape-size swelling. They seldom become inflamed or cause any problems other than cosmetic ones. Similar round swellings called *lipomas* appear on the body, usually the areas where there is subcutaneous fat in some abundance such as the hips, trunk, thigh or upper arms. They are solid benign tumours of fat, distinguishable by being soft, painless and freely mobile when palpated.

Malignant Tumours

There are only three skin cancers which are seen with any degree of frequency, and they are all becoming more frequent, partly because we expose ourselves more and more to the sun.

Melanomas in particular are five times as common as they were forty years ago and half of them arise in normal skin, the rest in moles. The first evidence is either a darkening in colour, itching, bleeding, spreading or ulceration and any of these symptoms should be viewed with suspicion as there is a risk of distant metastases occurring. Once the tumour has spread to the local lymph nodes only about one third of patients survive more than five years, especially if the original lesion is on the upper half of the body.

Epitheliomas or *squamous cell carcinomas* tend to arise on parts of the skin damaged by ultraviolet light, so they are common in places like Australia and South Africa among the white population and are usually seen on the face, ears, hands etc. They look like a small papule to begin with but soon ulcerate and bleed, growing more slowly than a melanoma and metastasizing later.

A somewhat similar appearance of ulceration on the face is seen in the *basal cell carcimoma*, more familiar as the *rodent ulcer*. Its name derives from its habit of destroying any tissue it meets locally and if left will grow extremely large, but it does not metastasize to other parts of the body. It is recognisable by its appearance being mostly in the elderly, its site on the cheek, nose or lip and its raised, rolled edge.

5

Bone: Disorders of Support

Bone is a living tissue and as such is constantly on the move in the sense that material is continually being deposited and removed, so that we renew our skeleton many times over in the course of our lifetime. It is not unlike fibreglass, in that it consists of a meshwork of fibres (collagen fibres) bound together with a resin (mucopolysaccharide polymers) and then hardened (with the minerals calcium and phosphorus). The rate at which the minerals are deposited and removed is undertaken by three hormones – *parathormone, calcitonin* and *vitamin D*. The regulation of the living 'matrix' of the bone is performed by three types of cells which create, preserve and destroy it (reminiscent of the Hindu trinity!) and are known as *osteoblasts, osteocytes* and *osteoclasts* respectively. Obviously these three have to operate in an integrated manner if health is to be maintained, and disease of bone is usually due either to an imbalance in their conduct or, much less commonly, to abnormalities of hormone production.

Development of Bone

During childhood minerals are deposited on pre-formed cartilage, a process called *ossification*, which is controlled by the osteoblasts at the *metaphysis* (see diagram 5.1), or more exactly the *epiphyseal line* of the metaphysis. If this area is injured by a fracture in childhood so that the epiphysis slips out of position (a *slipped epiphysis*), or is congenitally absent, then the bone will not elongate. It is the latter event which is seen in circus dwarfs and others who suffer from the congenital condition of *achondroplasia* (meaning 'no cartilaginous growth'), and are born with no functioning epiphyseal cartilage. Hence their limb bones remain short but the trunk and skull are relatively normal.

At the end of puberty growth of long bones terminates with the fusion of the epiphysis to prevent excessive height, but

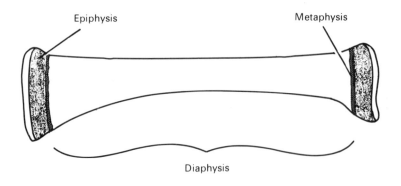

Fig. 5.1   *Anatomy of a long bone*

during the growth period of childhood some epiphyses are vulnerable to trauma, particularly the hip, the spine, the carpals of the wrist and the metatarsals in the feet. If the blood supply is temporarily suspended, e.g. from injury, the growing bone will soften for a while and may distort from pressure before hardening again. This process is named *osteochondritis* (juvenilis) and leads to local pain in the area affected, with stiffness if a joint is involved (usually the hip). Provided the softened bone is protected there is no distortion and no later disability but if, in the case of the hip, the child is allowed to walk, then later on osteoarthritis will set in. The different areas of the body where osteochondritis can occur are named after those who first described them, thus:

– *Perthe's disease* affects the hip to cause a limp and pain ('coxalgia').
– *Scheuermann's disease* affects the spine in adolescents and may cause pain and kyphosis.
– *Kienbock's disease* affects the lunate bone of the wrist.
– *Freiburg's disease* affects the head of the metatarsals and may cause pain on walking.

Rickets and Osteomalacia

Of the three hormones which regulate the mineral content of the bones vitamin D is the one which is usually missing, for the simple reason that it is the one which the body cannot always obtain (hence it is a 'vital amine' or vitamin). Normally vitamin D is obtained from animal fats in the diet or from the action of sunlight on skin, but may be missing in those whose diet is poor and who have little access to sunlight. Since during growth the majority of the activity of the bone-forming cells is at the epiphyseal line, it is here that any deficiencies in the deposition of minerals, for which vitamin D is responsible, will show up as swelling and softening in the form of *rickets*. These swellings are seen especially at the *wrists* and the *rib cartilages* where they resemble a necklace, the 'rickety rosary'. Although extremely rare in the West, rickets is still commonly seen in babies of underdeveloped countries.

Once the epiphyses have fused in adulthood then vitamin D deficiency has a more general effect on the bones and the skeleton becomes in effect demineralised, a condition called *osteomalacia*. As well as absence of vitamin D, lack of calcium in the blood will also have the effect of demineralising the bones, so osteomalacia may be a result of chronic renal failure losing calcium from the body or of adult coeliac disease preventing it from being absorbed. The classical cause of vitamin D lack may be seen sometimes in women in 'purdah' whose skin is never exposed to the sun, and especially at the time of pregnancy, when the demand is greatest, they may experience general aches and pains in the bones, and great weakness of the muscles (since calcium also plays a large part in enabling muscles to contract). In fact if the blood calcium should descend below a minimal level required by the muscles a form of spasm called *tetany* results (not to be confused with the infectious disease tetanus).

Osteoporosis

This is a much more common condition than osteomalacia (although the two are often confused), and all bones tend to develop osteoporosis with advancing age. They become less dense so that although the proportions of the ingredients – matrix and minerals alike – remain the same, there are less of them.

Although a natural process as old age approaches, osteoporosis is seen in the young under certain conditions such as immobilisation (e.g. after a fracture) and certain hormonal changes such as Cushing's disease, and following the menopause. Formation of bone matrix – the framework of the bone before minerals harden it – depends on a certain degree of physical stress being present as well as the necessary sex hormones to stimulate the osteoblasts to function. Thus menopausal women and the elderly of both sexes are mainly at risk and develop backache (the vertebrae are the most frequently affected bones) or even compression fractures and a stooping posture – the 'dowager's hump'. If the bones are even slightly stressed by a fall then they are liable to fracture at the weakest point, usually the wrist or neck of the femur. Lack of calcium does, however, play a significant part in osteoporosis as well as osteomalacia and it is important for the elderly to take sufficient calcium in the diet.

Fig. 5.2   *Typical posture of osteoporosis*

Scoliosis

The normal spine possesses a gentle curve convex at the shoulders and concave at the waist, and these are described as a dorsal *kyphosis* (Gr = stooping) and a lumbar *lordosis* (L = to praise) respectively.

However, the normal curves may become exaggerated as in osteoporosis or simply from a bad posture. Another type of abnormal curvature is when there is a sideways deviation or *scoliosis* (Gr = crooked), and this is seen in some teenagers, especially girls, as the spine develops. It is sometimes due to weakness of the muscles on one side as in polio, but more often there is no obvious cause.

Paget's Disease

Once again, this is a disorder of the normal balance between creation and destruction of bone, but in this case it is the osteoblasts which err on the side of creating more bone than is needed and in a somewhat irregular fashion, so that large cavities are left. These spaces are filled with very vascular fibrous tissue, and occupied by such a large volume of blood that eventually the patient may go into heart failure in the effort to maintain such a large circulation. The bones enlarge and distort as they expand, and the first part to be noticed may be the cranium when a larger hat is required. The long bones of the body also become bowed, thickened and irregular, hence the alternative name of 'osteitis deformans' for this condition, and the spine develops a kyphosis. Paget's disease is restricted to people over the age of 50 and is mild in most of them, perhaps even passing unnoticed unless the skull is Xrayed when increased density of bone is seen. In others it may give rise to pain and headaches from stretching of the periosteum, the pain being usually worse at night. In a small minority, about 1%, the osteoblasts get completely out of hand and become malignant after a few years.

6

Joints: Disorders of Stability

The terms 'arthritis' and 'rheumatism' are often used rather loosely to describe pains which are generally worse from movement, but strictly speaking the word 'arthritis' refers to pain coming from a joint, while 'rheumatism' means any ache or pain which moves about the body and therefore may emanate from muscles, tendons or ligaments. There are many diseases in which arthritis is part of the picture, but only about half a dozen or so are seen with any frequency.

Pain in a joint arises from the surfaces lining it – the cartilage or the synovium – and it is the latter which when inflamed will exude fluid into the joint and make it swell – the *effusion*. The cartilaginous surface of the joint is essentially for absorbing shocks to the bone and so has to withstand huge stresses on occasions. For example the knee joint has a surface area of approximately four square inches and transmits half of the weight of a 200 lb body, a pressure of about 25 lb/sq inch which is equal to that in a car tyre. On walking that pressure is doubled and on running quadrupled, so any excess weight that has to be carried puts it under great stress.

Osteoarthritis

The cartilage covering the bone is designed for a limited life and begins to wear out towards the end of the human lifespan in the joints which bear the most weight – the hip and knee especially. This process of wear in a joint is hastened if either the stress is excessive, usually because the person is overweight, or if it is applied at a slight angle and not through the centre of the joint, as may happen after a fracture, if the posture is poor, or where the joint is made unstable by some other form of arthritis such as rheumatoid arthritis. This process of physical wearing out or 'eburnation' of the cartilage is the basis of osteoarthritis, and as the cartilage is ground away the bone cells beneath frantically try to repair the damage by proliferating and mineralising the bone only to have it constantly cracked. Synovial fluid is squeezed into these cracked areas which develop tiny cysts called 'geodes' and this further weakens the bone. The only area where the proliferating bone is not being subjected to this pounding is at the very edges of the joint, and here irregular swellings called *osteophytes* grow, seen most clearly as *Heberden's nodes* in the fingers.

Primary osteoarthritis – that is the type occurring on account of age – is usually seen in the *spine, hips* and *knees* and is often accompanied by the process of osteoporosis which arrives simultaneously in middle age. When the intricate joints of the spine, particularly the facet joints, are afflicted by these ailments

Fig. 6.1   *Osteoarthritis of the hand*

the term *spondylosis* is used (Gr. spondylos = vertebra), and is the source of much backache in later life. Moreover, the osteophytes which develop in the neck have the habit of pressing on the vertebral arteries which run up inside the cervical vertebral bodies to supply the posterior parts of the cortex. This leads to neurological symptoms such as dizziness and loss of vision when the head is turned in a certain direction.

Not all joints affected by OA are painful, and it is not uncommon to see the hands painlessly involved, especially the joints indicated in diagram 6.1. If the carpometaphalangeal (CMP) joint at the base of the thumb is involved, however, then this is likely to be painful and quite incapacitating as it affects any activity involving gripping. Pain is also a common feature of OA of the hip, being worse on sudden movement especially going upstairs, and sometimes radiating down the thigh to the knee. If the knee is affected then it is likely to cause pain on walking over uneven ground or on descending the stairs. In all cases the pain is generally worse in cold, damp weather and remains constant during exercise, unlike that of rheumatoid arthritis which usually improves with movement.

Rheumatoid Arthritis

The disease gets its name from the word 'rheuma', meaning a stream of morbid humours flowing through the body, and refers to the widespread aches and pains which are often the earliest indicators that a general change is happening to the body. For it is not only the joints which are affected in RA and the term 'rheumatoid disease' is perhaps more appropriate to describe what is effectively a disorder of connective tissue of the joints, vessels, skin, lungs, eyes and lymphoid tissue.

There are many theories as to the origin of the condition, none of which are totally convincing, and they include infection, autoimmunity, genetic, food sensitivity and psychological. What has been established, however, is that in about 90% of cases an abnormal protein called *rheumatoid factor* is present in the blood. This is known to be an antibody against an antibody – the body appears to have seized one of its small IgG antibodies and made a much larger IgM antibody against it, and this larger antibody then goes on to attack the synovial membrane and other tissues. However, why this process should suddenly take place in about one person in 50 between the ages of 30–50 is very mysterious. One theory is that the proteins within the joints become damaged by infection or some other means and that this then alters their antigenic structure, making them no longer recognisable to the body which starts to make antibodies against them – an auto-immune disease.

The first signs of something amiss are often insidious and may include a fever, weakness and depression, weight loss or progressive morning stiffness of the hands, feet or knees. Occasionally the onset is sudden and dramatic with only one joint initially involved – a *monoarthritis* as opposed to the ensuing *polyarthritis*. The synovial membranes inflame and secrete fluid into the joint which swells up and becomes extremely tender and stiff during the acute phase. Later the synovium proliferates and thickens (in contrast to OA) to produce what is called a *pannus* (L. = cloak), and if the joint is not mobilised then there is a risk that the two synovial membranes will fuse and produce an immobile, useless joint. It is this pannus which causes the persistant pain, stiffness and limited range of movement in affected joints (and which is removed in the operation of synovectomy).

However the condition starts, it is likely to progress to a polyarthritis, where several joints are affected though not necessarily severely, and these are commonly the hands, which are a prime target. They develop characteristic swelling of the knuckles which deviate towards the ulna, and of the proximal interphalangeal joints (finger joints nearest the knuckles) which develop a spindle shape and sometimes the characteristic *swan neck deformity* of the fingers or the *Z deformity* of the thumbs.

As well as the hands, any synovial joint may be involved, and especially the wrists, elbows, shoulders, knees and feet, less commonly the hips, ankles and spine. The same joints are involved in the feet as in the hands, and give the sensation of walking on pebbles in bare feet as the metatarsals are unstable, requiring special shoes. If the knees are involved there is wasting of the quadriceps muscle of the thigh and a *Baker's cyst* may emerge from the rear of the joint as a soft swelling of the weak point of the joint capsule, and possibly even rupture into the muscles of the calf to simulate a deep vein thrombosis.

Involvement of the cervical spine is not infrequent and gives rise to pain in the upper part of the neck. Where the atlanto-axial joint is involved there is the possibility of dangerous instability of the odontoid peg where it passes through the atlas and may subluxate (partially dislocate) to press on the cord, so patients complaining of pains running up to the scalp should be treated with circumspection.

Spindle-shaped swelling

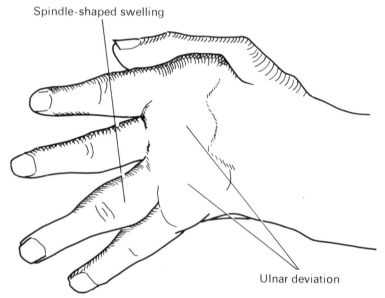

Ulnar deviation

Fig. 6.2   *Advanced rheumatoid arthritis of the hand*

Non Articular Manifestations.

Many other body systems may be involved in RA, some of which are rare and will not be discussed. One of the more common is the *subcutaneous nodule* seen on the bony prominences of the elbows, shoulders and knees or the tendons of the wrists and feet. They are hard, painless swellings of degenerating connective tissue, up to 1″ in diameter, formed in response to leakage of the rheumatoid factor from damaged vessels. Another common concomitant of RA is *anaemia* which arises because the marrow is inhibited from taking up iron (although there is no shortage in the body), and this and the thinning of the skin which occurs gives the patient a pale complexion. Some cases of anaemia are made worse by gastric bleeding from aspirin and other drugs taken for the arthritis.

The *lymph nodes* are sometimes enlarged, often in the neighbourhood of a badly affected joint, and this is especially seen in children who have a slightly different form of RA known as *Still's disease* which includes general swelling of the lymph glands and spleen.

Another fairly frequent consequence is the drying up of the secretions of the salivary and the tear glands, leading to difficulty swallowing and sore eyes. The condition is termed *Sjogren's syndrome*.

The appearance of breathlessness in especially men with RA may indicate that the pleura has become involved and has reacted by forming a *pleural effusion*. Women are more likely to notice compression of the median nerve in the wrist and feel tingling sensations in the hands – the *carpal tunnel syndrome*.

Crystal Deposition and Gout

Despite its music hall image gout is one of the most painful conditions known to man (women are generally immune until after the menopause), and was well described by Hippocrates. Pitt the Elder suffered severely from gout all his life and had to be wheeled about in a specially constructed chair, which has perhaps encouraged the view that it is a disease of retired colonels brought on by high living. In fact the average sufferer of gout is a young man in his 20s or 30s who develops intermittent pains at the base of his big toe which are easily ascribed to strain or injury until they flare up and the joint becomes hot, red and swollen ('podagra').

The problem is one of uric acid crystals forming in the joints and other places, usually because the amount in the blood is excessive. Uric acid is made from DNA and RNA, the constituents of the nuclei of the cells, and these are broken down in the liver and passed to the blood for excretion. The amount which the kidney can excrete is limited, and if this level is exceeded then the 'pool' builds up and some of it crystallises in the joints, the kidney or the cartilage (the latter known as *tophi*). The preferred joint is the *metatarsophalangeal* (MTP) joint of the toe (see figure 6.3), perhaps because it is the lowest, or the coldest, in the body. Sometimes other joints in the body become affected, particularly the knee and elbow, and develop excruciating pain on movement or touch.

If uric acid crystals are formed very rapidly by the body then they may occur as *stones in the kidney* or even crystallise in the tubules and lead to renal failure, although this is rare. Tophaceous deposits are seen in longstanding gouty subjects and occupy the pinna of the ears and the tendons of the arms, where they may eventually ulcerate and exude chalky material (L. tofus = rock).

Gout tends to run in families, and after a first attack there may be no further ones, or they may be few and far between. It is worth avoiding rich foods such as red meat and dairy products as far as possible, as this is often successful in preventing further attacks. Such attacks may sometimes be precipitated by diuretics, when the fluid level of the body drops and effectively increases the uric acid in the blood, or if the body is breaking down an excessive number of cells as in leukaemia or psoriasis.

Uric acid is not the only substance to crystallise out in the joints, however, and elderly people are sometimes liable to what is known as 'pseudogout'. In this much less painful condition the large joints, especially the knees, are affected and the mineral in question is a calcium salt, calcium pyrophosphate. The joints do become severely disrupted, however, and this may later lead to osteoarthritis.

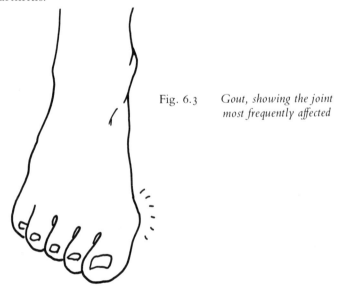

Fig. 6.3   *Gout, showing the joint most frequently affected*

Ankylosing Spondylitis

The joint pathology we have been looking at so far is confined to the synovial joints, those containing fluid and designed for greater movement than the more limited cartilaginous joints. These are seen in the spine linking the vertebrae, and in the ribs and sternum where large movements are not needed, so the elasticity of the cartilage will suffice. Unfortunately these joints too are not without their problems on occasions, and are liable to calcification and even eventually ossification when the cartilage is replaced by bony tissue. If that happens then no movement is possible and the joint is said to be *ankylosed*.

Since the word for spinal arthritis is 'spondylitis', the disease of *ankylosing spondylitis* indicates stiffening of the spine, and that is the main long-term effect of the condition. It comes about by gradual ossification of the intervertebral discs, but the earliest signs are in either the *sacro-iliac joints* or in the periphery of the body where the cartilaginous tendons are inserted into the bone (the 'entheses'). The favoured entheses where calcification takes place are the sole of the foot in the plantar fascia (*plantar fasciitis*), the Achilles tendon (tendinitis), the hip bones and the shoulder girdle, and these will all be tender on palpation. The classic site for AS, however, is the sacroiliac joint which becomes progressively fused and stiff and usually heralds the onset of the condition.

The story is one of stiffness and aching in the lower back on waking in the mornings, usually in a young man, and the pain eases with movement only to recur on sitting for long periods during the day. There is also a feeling of progressive, inexplicable weakness and fatigue in some, who may be suspected as malingering until the other symptoms make themselves known. Gradually the flexibility of the spine is lost, especially if mobilisation exercises are not encouraged, and much damage is done by resting (as used to happen). This leads to rapid spinal rigidity with swollen, calcified discs – the *bamboo spine* – so called because of its similarity on Xray to a stem of bamboo. Men are far more likely than women to be affected by this disease, often in their adolescence or early adult life, and some of them will go on to develop complications. These include an *iritis* and take the form of a sore, red eye, or less commonly damage to the aorta and the aortic valve.

Reiter's Syndrome

This form of arthritis is an occasional complication of either diarrhoea or urethritis, coming on 3–4 weeks after the acute episode and affecting the large synovial joints and sometimes cartilaginous joints as well. Reiter's original description was a triad composed of *arthritis, urethritis* and *iritis or conjunctivitis,* but sometimes skin rashes may also occur. A similar type of reactive arthritis may occur in those who suffer from ulcerative colitis or Crohn's disease.

7

Muscles and Soft Tissues: Disorders of Movement

The muscles of the body form a system of levers which operate the joints and in most cases span the joint either alone or with the aid of a tendon. Trauma or overuse can easily damage either the muscle or its tendon, and in the case of the latter this is particularly serious as it is much less vascular and takes far longer to heal. A pulled muscle indicates that some of the fibres are torn, usually on account of violent or unaccustomed exercise, and until the bleeding has been absorbed using the muscle will be painful. Sometimes pain arises spontaneously in a muscle which goes into spasm in certain areas which become tender and swollen as *fibrositis*. This happens especially in the large muscles of the lower back and is termed *lumbago*.

Ligaments, which connect bone to bone and stabilise the joints, are liable to *sprain* if excess force is used on a joint, and although they are elastic, if the sprain is severe the ligament is left stretched and swollen. The immediate treatment of one of these sprains is to apply a cold compress with a crepe bandage and rest the limb by elevating it to reduce swelling. If the joint itself is damaged then the muscles which operate it will tend to atrophy unless exercised, and rehabilitation plays a large part in such injuries. Actual paralysis or weakness of a muscle is almost always due to neurological problems, apart from the rare congenital muscular dystrophies and myasthenia gravis.

Because of the complex interaction of muscles, tendons, joints and ligaments it is preferable to depart for a while from the systems approach and look at the soft tissues in various areas of the body individually.

The Spine

Unlike the limbs, the spine is not a lever. This may appear to be stating the obvious but many of the problems which the back incurs arise from using it as if it were. Nature designed the spine for both support and flexibility, and did so by wedging it in the pelvis at the sacroiliac joints and then 'guying' it with muscles. It is when these muscles are not properly used or become slack that the intervertebral joints and discs develop displacements which may lead to pressure on the nerve roots as they emerge from the spine. If they are compressed then the person experiences referred pain in the area supplied by the nerve and may additionally notice weakness of the muscles. The nerves supplying the arm and the leg are most likely to be affected and the pain is termed *brachial neuralgia* or *sciatica* respectively.

The Shoulder

Nature had to compromise on the stability of the shoulder joint in order to maximise the range of movements available to the

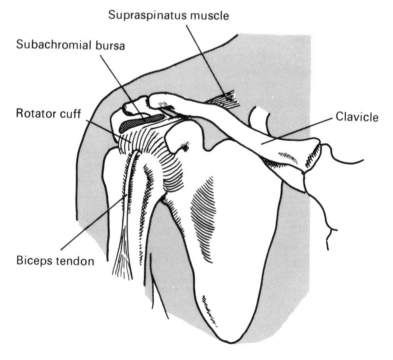

Supraspinatus muscle

Subachromial bursa

Rotator cuff

Clavicle

Biceps tendon

Fig. 7.1   *The shoulder*

arm, and did so by making the socket in the scapula rather shallow which allows the shoulder to dislocate downwards very easily. Compensation for the lack of bony protection comes in the form of a ring of muscles and ligaments which grip the head of the humerus firmly like a 'lions claw' and form the *rotator cuff*, and when this is torn or damaged the shoulder sustains pain on the least movement in any direction – the *frozen shoulder*. This may come on spontaneously or follow an injury, and as the pain gradually lessens so the stiffness increases and may limit movements for many months unless adequate therapy is forthcoming.

If, however, inflammation is limited to one of the muscles or tendons running over the joint then only the movements initiated by that muscle are painful. Thus *bicipital tendonitis* will cause pain on flexion of the joint, where the biceps tendon runs over the front of it, and *supraspinatus tendonitis* pain on abduction (movement away from the body). A similar pain on abducting the joint is found when the subachromial bursa is inflamed. This is a form of bursitis caused by a blow or pressure to the outside of the shoulder, and pain is only found as the arm comes up to the horizontal, the remainder of the arc being pain free.

The shoulder may also be affected by any condition damaging the sympathetic nerve supply of the region, particularly a stroke, myocardial infarction or cervical spondylosis. This can reduce the blood flow to the shoulder and hand together, and the two become cold and atrophied – the *shoulder-hand syndrome*.

The Elbow

This is a hinge joint between the ulna and the humerus, and also contains a pivot between the head of the radius and the ulna to allow the forearm to pronate and supinate. The annular ligament retaining the head of the radius in position is relatively weak in young children, so that a sudden jerk on their hand may pull the radial head through the ligament (*pulled elbow*). The hand will then be held pronated across the body until the radius is replaced by firm pressure with supination which 'screws' the head back into place.

The olecranon process at the back of the elbow is protected by a bursa which may become inflamed in someone who spends a lot of time leaning on their elbows, such as a student. This swells up into an *olecranon bursitis* the size of a golf ball for a few days, but usually disappears with rest. Just above the capitulum of the humerus (see figure 7.2) ·is the origin of the forearm abductor muscles which operate the wrist. You can feel this on yourself by folding your arms, when the little finger of your right hand will lie over the point, and if you now abduct your hand at the wrist you will feel the tendon contract. It is tendinitis at this exact location, caused by overuse of the wrist in hammering, sawing or even tennis, which is known as *tennis elbow*. A similar tendinitis on the medial side is called *golfer's elbow*.

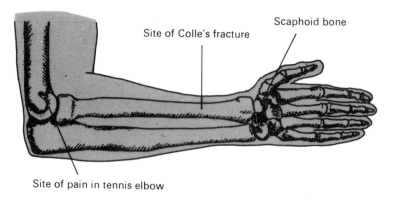

Fig. 7.2   *The elbow and hand*

The Wrist and Hand

Many of the movements in this area are performed by muscles located in the forearms and operating by long tendons which run across the wrist and into the hand. This exposes the joint to sprains and fractures, as well as inflammation of the tendon sheaths (*tenosynovitis*). In the latter condition the synovial sheath covering the tendon becomes inflamed from overuse and swells, pinching the tendon and making it difficult to use as well as painful. If this happens to the tendon supplying the finger flexors, then it may be difficult to straighten the finger after flexion (*trigger finger*). When it occurs in the abductor tendons to the thumb it is sometimes called *de Quervain's syndrome*, and may be a symptom of rheumatoid arthritis.

A more common condition is that known as *Dupuytren's*

contracture, which is a thickening of the tendons which run across the palm of the hand, especially those supplying the little and ring fingers. This causes painless shortening and consequent flexion of the fingers which weakens the grip. It tends to be a familial complaint, but is also more common in those who have epilepsy or alcoholism.

Fig. 7.3   *Dupuytren's contracture*

A fall on the outstretched hand is likely to cause a fracture in the locality, either a *Colle's fracture* of the ulna in the elderly, with its typical 'dinner fork' displacement, or a *scaphoid fracture* in the young, with tenderness in the 'anatomical snuffbox' when it is pinched. Because of the large number of tiny carpal bones in the wrist and the joints between them, swellings of synovial membrane may extrude from the joints in the area and form what are known (inaccurately) as *ganglia*. They are painless and nothing more than unsightly, but it is not recommended that they be ruptured, either by the family bible or anything else.

The anterior aspect of the wrist is covered by a band of fibrous tissue which guides the flexor tendons and the median nerve through the carpal tunnel beneath. If damaged by trauma or arthritis, or if the underlying tissues swell from oedema or myxoedema, the resultant pressure on the nerve will lead to pain, tingling and weakness of the fingers, particularly at night, the well known *carpal tunnel syndrome*. Many individuals with no overt pathology suffer from this condition, and a useful test is gently to extend the wrist which brings on the symptoms.

Fig. 7.4   *Ganglion*

The Knee

This is a hinge joint and somewhat vulnerable as it is unprotected by muscle tissue. Moreover it has to transmit some truly enormous strains through the tendons which cross it, and relies heavily on ligaments to keep the joint surfaces in place. As well as the articular cartilage common to all synovial joints, the tibial surface possesses two thick pads called menisci, semilunar cartilages which act as additional shock absorbers. These are liable to tear if the knee is flexed to a right angle and then twisted, as happens often in football or mining injuries, when the condyle which protrudes from the femur will grind it into the tibia and tear it. These torn menisci will then flap about and jam in the joint when it bends, leading to locking, the main symptom. If the stresses to the knee come from the side or the front, then the supporting ligaments which join the bones are liable to be stretched and torn, leading to local tenderness and swelling of the joint. This *effusion* into the joint happens because some of the ligaments actually run inside the joint capsule.

The most important structures supporting the knee, however, are the muscles, especially the quadriceps muscle which is inserted into the tibia at the front, via the patella, and extends the knee (see figure 7.5). This muscle makes up the bulk of the front of the thigh and if it becomes weakened from damage or disuse then the knee may suddenly give way, as happens particularly in the elderly after they have been ill in bed for some time. It may also occur in teenage girls whose patellar bones may click as they drift laterally across the joint as they walk, known as *chondromalacia patellae*. The remedy is to exercise and tighten the muscles by building them up.

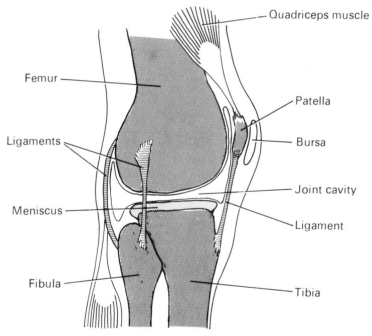

Fig. 7.5   *The knee*

The Ankle and Foot

The ankle is a hinge joint in between a mortice formed by the malleoli of the fibula and tibia, and has little sideways movement except when the toes are pointed. Consequently you are more likely to sprain or even fracture your ankle (*Pott's fracture*) if you walk heavily on your heels rather than your toes on rough ground. The main supports for the ankle are the strong medial and lateral ligaments which are stretched if the foot is forcibly over-adducted or abducted, usually the former. Thus the commonest sprain of the ankle is an *inversion sprain* with tenderness and swelling over the lateral ligament. If there is tenderness of the lateral malleolus then suspect a fracture of the lower end of the fibula.

At the back of the ankle the Achilles tendon is inserted into the calcaneus, and pain in this area may be due to a tendinitis with inflammation and swelling of the tendon sheath directly behind the ankle. Careful palpation will usually elicit *crepitus*, a slight grating sensation on movement, and this usually occurs from overuse. On occasions the tendon may even rupture during sudden exertion and there will be a palpable gap. Sometimes the pain is felt lower down over the back of the calcaneus, at the point of insertion of the tendon where a bursa is located, which signifies a *calcaneal bursitis*.

At the front of the bottom of the calcaneum, on the sole of the foot, are inserted the plantar muscles via the plantar fascia, which maintain the arch and spring of the foot. The tendon at this point may calcify and produce a painful *plantar fasciitis*, so the patient develops a limp as he cannot bear weight on this area. This happens in those who have overstretched, poorly-developed arches and do a lot of running; it may in some cases be a sign of ankylosing spondylitis or Reiter's syndrome.

The sole of the foot may also give rise to pain further forward, over the heads of the metatarsal bones and therefore called *metatarsalgia*. Again this may be due to running on hard surfaces in inappropriate shoes, as the first metatarsophalangeal (MTP) joint is very susceptible to trauma and easily becomes stiff and immobile so is given the name *hallux rigidus*. Later this may develop into osteoarthritis of the joint and be confused with gout which has a predilection for the same joint but is far more tender. *Stress fractures* are also common in the metatarsal bones and present with forefoot pain and a limp after severe excercise. They are easily missed as the hairline fracture does not show up on an Xray until callus has formed several days later.

A very common condition of the feet is *hallux valgus* or

hammer toes, which tend to be constitutional and run in families. The deformity consists of a 'valgus' or abduction of the MTP joint of the big toe or hallux. This usually develops a large bursa over it known as a *bunion* which becomes inflamed and painful. The second and third toes then become hooked over the hallux and are known as 'claw toes', and these gradually subluxate and lead to instability of the foot with the passage of time.

Fig. 7.6   *A. Hallux valgus, B. Claw toes*

Hernias

One of the main functions of the abdominal muscles is to contain the viscera and keep the organs in position. On occasions they either become too weak or have excess pressure exerted on them, and so a gap appears between the fibres allowing the abdominal organs to partially or completely protrude, this protrusion being a *hernia.* The hernial sac is likely to bulge through in places where there is a potential weakness in the abdominal muscles such as the groin or the diaphragm, often at the site where other structures penetrate the wall. Once the musculature has started to give it is seldom possible to strengthen it by exercises, and the tendency is for the bulge gradually to increase in size as the months go by.

If the hernia goes back inside the abdomen on relaxation or lying down, or can easily be pushed back, then it is said to be *reducible,* but if not then it is *irreducible* and is then at risk of strangulation or obstruction. When a hernia *strangulates* then the blood supply, which accompanies the loop of bowel, is cut off and the bowel begins to die and eventually will become gangrenous if left for longer than about 6–8 hours. *Obstruction* of a hernia means that the contents of the intestine cannot move through it, so there are a series of colicky pains as the pressure builds up. Normally, apart from a heavy, dragging sensation a hernia is painless unless one of these complications occurs, so any pain indicates that intervention is urgently needed.

Inguinal Hernia

This type of hernia is mostly seen in men or boys and is due to the fact that when the testis descends into the scrotum it travels down the inguinal canal in between two layers of muscle in the groin. The entrance to the canal (internal ring) is half an inch above the femoral pulse in the groin, and the exit, the external ring, is in the top of the scrotum where it can be palpated, and it is here that the hernia will emerge. Sometimes it can be seen rolling down the inguinal canal when the subject coughs, and a finger over the internal ring will prevent this. This, of course, is the function of a truss, the type of padded belt worn by those who are unfit for an operation to sew up the hernia ('herniorrhaphy').

Occasionally women get inguinal hernias, but in their case the swelling does not go indirectly down the inguinal canal but pushes directly through the weak abdominal wall at the level of the external ring, and this can be proved by the fact that its emergence cannot be prevented by pressure over the internal ring.

Femoral Hernia

Because women have a wider pelvis than men the potential space under the inguinal ligament, through which all the vessels and nerves leave for the leg, is much greater, as everything is less packed together. It is down this femoral canal below the inguinal ligament that a hernia may develop, and this can occasionally occur in men in whom the risk of strangulation is high because the aperture is so much smaller.

Umbilical Hernia

These are commonly seen in newborn babies as a soft bulge

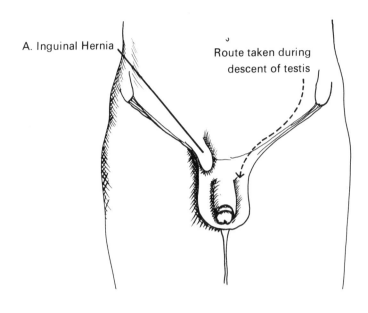

A. Inguinal Hernia

Route taken during descent of testis

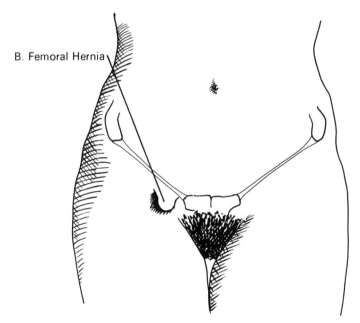

B. Femoral Hernia

Fig. 7.7   *Hernias in men and women*

around the umbilicus, and swell up when the baby cries. They reduce very easily and so there is no risk of strangulation, in fact they only exist because the muscles have not yet developed and almost always disappear within two years. A similar hernia may be seen in women after pregnancy but in this case the swelling is just above the umbilicus and is therefore known as a para-umbilical hernia, and seldom resolves spontaneously.

Incisional Hernia

After a midline abdominal operation or *laparotomy* (Gr. laparos = soft) the muscles are sewn together but never with the original strength so if there is a cough and the intra-abdominal pressure is elevated, or if the wound becomes infected and the tissues break down, the intestines may herniate through and form a large bulge under the skin. This is very unsightly but seldom dangerous and can usually be repaired.

Hiatus Hernia

These are herniations of the stomach through the diaphragm and are covered in Chapter 12.

8

Blood: Disorders of Transport

The blood which circulates in virtually all our tissues is made up of cells and plasma which each contribute about half the volume. In the event of a serious haemorrhage both, of course, are lost but the body is able to make up the plasma within a matter of hours since this is composed mainly of water. The cellular component takes a little longer, however, and during this time we are depleted of red and white cells and are slightly anaemic. Because of the huge rate at which the marrow can produce red cells (if layed edge to edge the daily output would stretch from London to Edinburgh), the anaemia only becomes significant if we continue to lose blood from, say, heavy periods or bleeding piles at a rate faster than the body can produce them. In order for this production line to operate with efficiency there must be no shortage of raw materials, and that means protein, vitamin B12, folic acid and, of course, iron.

Iron Deficiency Anaemia

The oxygen carrying ability of the red cell is due to the unique properties of haemoglobin, the iron-containing red pigment of which it is composed, and in making this the body uses in its lifetime enough iron to make a six inch nail. This iron has to come from our food, so any dietary deficiency will affect production, as will any problems with absorbing it by the gut. Delayed weaning in babies may cause iron deficiency as there is very little iron present in milk. Iron must first be acidified in the stomach before going on to be absorbed by the small intestine, so any operation which removes the acid-secreting part of the stomach such as a *partial gastrectomy* will affect absorption, and so will conditions such as coeliac disease which damages the jejunum. Once inside the body the iron is stored for future needs in the liver.

The most common reason for iron deficiency is simply that there is a continuous loss of blood, either from heavy periods or from somewhere in the gut. So-called *occult bleeding* may feature with peptic ulcer, aspirin or other anti-arthritic drugs, cirrhosis of the liver or sometimes it is the first sign of a carcinoma of the stomach. The amount of blood lost daily is not enough to be detectable as melaena in the stools, but over the months it adds up to a significant amount. Sometimes patients have adequate iron reserves in the body but are unable to use them because the marrow is affected by some deep-seated disease like renal failure or rheumatoid arthritis, in which case giving iron does not help much.

If the marrow is starved of iron it responds by putting less haemoglobin into each erythrocyte, so the cells become slightly pale (*hypochromic*). It also makes each cell slightly smaller than usual, these being termed *microcytes*, and these two features are diagnostic of iron deficiency anaemia when seen in the red blood cells.

The early features of iron deficiency are quite subtle and include weariness and fatigue, anorexia and poor resistance to infection. In children the desire for strange substances such as coal or chalk may be the first sign, known as *pica* (L = magpie). Later, the mucus membranes look pale, the tongue becomes smooth and sore with *glossitis* and the nails crack and become brittle and *spoon-shaped*. Finally there is breathlessness, insomnia, palpitations, angina and difficulty swallowing in some, although many of these symptoms are common and not necessarily due to anaemia. In time of doubt an estimate of the haemoglobin content of the blood and the discovery of hypochromic microcytes will confirm the diagnosis.

Pernicious Anaemia

For many years it had been known that in middle age some people quite suddenly began to develop *indigestion* and *glossitis* with a sore tongue and cracked lips, and then a year or so later became very pale and slightly *jaundiced*, finally succumbing to a form of *paralysis*. So resistant was the condition to treatment of any kind that it was known as 'pernicious anaemia', and it was Addison who first observed the connection between the stomach and the anaemia, and whose name is still attached to the disease. However, it was not until 1954 that the role of *intrinsic factor* from the peptic cells of the stomach was finally established as being necessary to bind the B12 and enable it to be absorbed in the small intestine.

Pernicious anaemia is very seldom due to dietary deficiency as the body only requires minute amounts of vitamin B12 and has a large store of it in the liver which lasts several years. In some people, however, the peptic cells of the stomach atrophy around the age of 40–60, and this is usually due to an autoimmune process, so *antibodies to the gastric cells* are found in the blood. This tendency is inherited, and the individuals are typically fair and blue-eyed but with a lemon tinge to the skin on account of the mild jaundice.

Vitamin B12 contains the element cobalt and is essential for the construction of the wall of the erythrocyte in the marrow, as well as maintaining the well-being of the myelin sheath of the nerves of the spinal cord. If this vitamin is not available the cell wall is thin and fragile and breaks down prematurely to release excess bilirubin into the blood. The cells also end up a size too large and are termed *macrocytes* or, when immature, *megaloblasts*, in contrast to the microcytes of iron deficiency. If diagnosis of the condition is delayed, the spinal cord will start to *demyelinate* causing tingling, weakness and loss of reflexes in the feet and legs, followed eventually by similar damage to the brain in the form of *dementia*. Because the problem is essentially one of deficiency it is eminently treatable by giving B12 by injection (to by-pass the absent intrinsic factor), but any neurological damage already sustained unfortunately cannot be repaired.

Folic acid, so called because it was first obtained from foliage, is another B vitamin required for the construction of mature erythrocytes. It is present in adequate amounts in most diets, but *pregnancy* makes heavy demands on the body's reserves and supplements may be needed. If they are not forthcoming then the marrow makes the larger megaloblasts and these work less efficiently, but deficiency of this vitamin does not lead to the neurological consequences of B12 deficiency.

Haemolytic Anaemias – Sickle Cell and Thalassaemia

Not all anaemia is due to a deficiency in production of cells, some types of anaemia are caused by premature breakdown of the erythrocyte before its allotted time span (about 120 days), a process called *haemolysis*. This leads to the liberation of large amounts of iron which is retained for further use, as well as the formation of quantities of bilirubin which is carried to the liver for use in the bile and leads to a degree of jaundice in the body (the megaloblastic anaemias are also examples of this as we have seen). The increase in turnover only becomes a problem if the breakdown of cells exceeds the regenerative capacity of the marrow when a *haemolytic crisis* occurs against a background of haemolytic anaemia.

Most haemolytic anaemias are inherited defects of red cell stability, either because the envelope of the cell is the wrong shape (*spherocytosis*) or because the haemoglobin within is abnormal in some way (*haemoglobinopathy*). It is the latter which is responsible for the two conditions of *thalassaemia* and *sickle cell anaemia*.

Normal haemoglobin consists of a four-armed structure, each arm containing an atom of iron and a chain of about 150 amino acids coiled around it. The four arms are arranged in two pairs with two identical alpha chains on one side and two beta chains on the other. The exact nature and sequence of the amino acids in the chain is determined genetically and of critical importance to the successful functioning of the molecule, so when they are incorrect the result is that less oxygen can be carried and the cell wall may also collapse.

Sickle cell anaemia is one such inherited condition found only among those of black African descent. It is likely that the disease has persisted throughout generations because of the significant protection the abnormal haemoglobin gives against malaria. One or both of the side chains of the molecule contains substituted amino acids and this leads to the *trait* or the *disease* respectively. In the case of sickle cell trait there is little evidence of anaemia, and it is only the presence of two abnormal side chains which leads to real problems in the form of sickle cell disease, inherited from two parents with the trait. Here the anaemia is severe and comes on a few months after birth, when many of the children die. Those who survive develop an *enlarged liver and spleen* to cope with the increasing turnover and their lives are punctuated with severe *bone pains* when a haemolytic crisis occurs and the tissue is deprived of blood and dies.

Thalassaemia inherits its name from the occurrence in races which inhabit the Mediterranean shores (Gr. thalassa = sea), although it is also widespread in parts of Asia. There is reluctance on the part of the marrow to synthesize adequate amounts of adult haemoglobin, so that which is used is mostly of the foetal type and therefore rapidly destroyed. Foetal haemoglobin is of a slightly different specification for use in the uterus and is normally discarded soon after birth and adult haemoglobin substituted (hence the incidence of a degree of jaundice in most babies at the time of birth).

Where it persists to only a slight degree the condition of *thalassaemia minor* is said to occur and, like the sickle cell trait, there is little actual disability. *Thalassaemia major* entails severe anaemia with the marrow enlarging as it struggles to maintain supplies, causing prominence of the bones of the skull and face as well as hypertrophy of the liver and spleen to dispose of the breakdown products (indeed the spleen is often surgically removed in an attempt to slow down the process of destruction).

Polycythaemia

This condition of too many red cells in the circulation is found under normal physiological conditions in those living at high altitude when the low oxygen content of the air stimulates the marrow. An analagous situation may happen in the event of *chronic respiratory disease* when there is less oxygen in the blood and a similar stimulus is evoked.

However in the condition of *primary polycythaemia* there is an apparently unprovoked increase in the quantity of erythrocytes in the blood which may reach large numbers and cause an increase in the viscosity, slowing down the circulation and encouraging the blood to clot in the veins. Earlier symptoms are headaches and dizziness, itching of the skin and a flushed face. The blood pressure is elevated and the congestion leads sometimes to bleeding or menorrhagia, so that it may be necessary to remove a pint of blood from the circulation every few weeks. The cause of the disease is not known, but some cases go on to develop a form of leukaemia after many years.

White Cell Disorders

The white cells circulating in the blood are mainly *granulocytes* (also called *myelocytes* from the Greek word myelos meaning marrow), *lymphocytes* and a few *monocytes*. However there are many other white cells in the lymphatic system in the form of *lymphocytes*, and disorders of these stationary white cells, such as *lymphoma* and *myeloma* were discusssed in Chapter 2. Unlike erythrocytes, the leucocytes are only very rarely depleted in a condition called *agranulocytosis*, when the marrow stops producing them because of suppression by drugs or infection. More commonly, though still only affecting about 1 person in 10,000, the marrow overproduces either lymphocytes or myelocytes (granulocytes) in the condition of leukaemia.

Leukaemia

The number of white cells produced by the marrow varies widely and may suddenly increase in the presence of infection, so the marrow may be called upon to work overtime. All the different types of cells in the blood derive ultimately from a single type of cell in the marrow called the *stem cell* by a process of differentiation followed by maturation, and during the maturation process the early cells are termed 'blast' forms (Gr. blasto = bud), as illustrated in figure 8.1. Leukaemia is a form of cancer caused by the uncontrolled multiplication of a single one of these white cells at some stage in its process of maturation, and the symptoms of the disease picture therefore differ according to how mature or primitive that leucocyte was when it began to get out of control.

Thus *acute lymphatic leukaemia* is a form of leukaemia affecting the lymphatic cells at an early stage of maturation when they are still lymphoblasts and the leukaemic cell is quite primitive and undifferentiated and therefore more destructive. This means that it is a sudden, acute condition and is seen in young children in whom huge numbers of ineffectual lymphoblasts in the marrow crowd out the production of erythrocytes and thrombocytes as

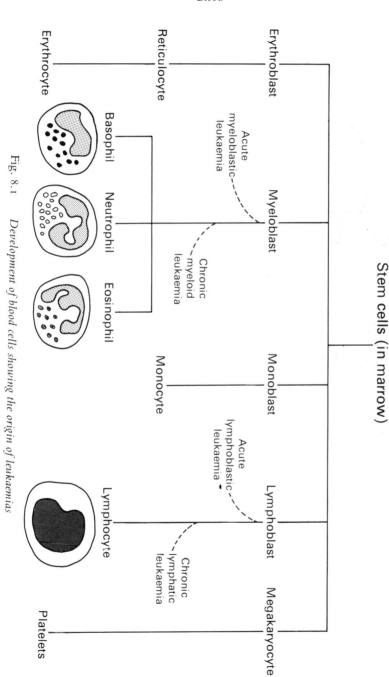

Fig. 8.1   *Development of blood cells showing the origin of leukaemias*

well as the other white cell series. This leads to the symptoms of *anaemia* and *pallor, bruising* and *bleeding gums* and *recurrent infections* such as sore throats and pneumonia. The lymphocytes occupy not only the blood but also the lymph nodes causing them to swell, as well as enlarging the liver and spleen.

Acute myeloid leukaemia involves people of a much older age group, usually those over 60, and is a rarer disease. Many of the symptoms are similar to those of acute lymphoblastic leukaemia, but there is less swelling of the lymphatic tissue. Because no effective neutrophils are available *infections* set in early and can be rampant, sometimes overwhelming the patient before the diagnosis is made.

Chronic lymphatic and *chronic myeloid leukaemia* are altogether slower processes whereby the cells produced, though malignant, are very much more mature and thus go some way to serving the needs of the body. It may be a matter of years rather than weeks before the symptoms become apparent and the condition diagnosed, and they happen very gradually. The sufferer is usually an elderly person and the anaemia, lymphatic enlarge-ment and general ill-health pass unnoticed for a while. They may develop night sweats and weight loss, culminating in an infection, and the disease smoulders on for many years before finally gathering pace and changing to the acute type of leukaemia.

Clotting Disorders

Blood clotting is a complex process involving a number of chemical and cellular chain reactions before the clot is finally formed. In many patients coagulation may occur too readily and lead to a thrombosis in a vital vessel and such people are often treated with *anticoagulant drugs* such as Warfarin to slow this process down. Because it is vital that some clotting ability is retained periodic checks of their 'clotting time' must be made and the dose adjusted if necessary.

It is possible on rare occasions for one of these clotting factors to be absent, and this defect is inherited. One such is *haemophilia* which, though rare, is perhaps the best known. This particular disorder affects only men, being inherited on the sex chromo-some, and in those who have it there is extensive bleeding after a cut and large *ecchymoses* after minor trauma. Sometimes bleeding occurs internally, especially into the joints which become damaged and arthritic in adulthood. The missing *factor VIII* is given by regular transfusion, and more severe injuries treated with additional injections which must be kept to hand.

Thrombocytopenia, or lack of sufficient thrombocytes in the blood, leads eventually to a similar situation of bleeding after trauma, but usually there is earlier evidence that the number of thrombocytes are falling and this takes the form of widespread *petechiae* in the skin. The falling count is due to widespread self-destruction of blood platelets by an auto-immune process, resulting either spontaneously (*idiopathic thrombocytopenic purpura*) or after certain drugs.

9

Heart: Disorders of Propulsion

The heart is more than a pump, it is often thought of as the seat of the emotions and intimately related to our feelings. We speak of someone as warm-hearted or stony-hearted, in grief our hearts break and in fear or excitement they miss a beat. Because of this intimate awareness of our heart there is often a concern about heart disease and this may create actual symptoms in the form of pain, palpitations and difficulty breathing. Unfortunately these symptoms can mimic those caused by the major cause of death in the UK, *coronary artery disease*, so the fears are sometimes justifiable. Since the turn of the century there has been a steady increase of heart attacks in the West, until the last 10 years or so when the statistics have begun to improve. At present they account for one third of male deaths and one quarter of those in women, exceeding all other causes of death including cancer.

The Pathology of Coronary Heart Disease

By the early teens most of us have already developed the very earliest evidence of narrowing of the arteries which starts as deposits of white, fatty streaks of cholesterol on the intimal layer of the major arteries. Over the years, at a rate largely in accordance with the factors listed below, these streaks may mature into thickened *plaques* which project into the lumen of the vessel and narrow it, reducing the circulation to a trickle. Eventually the plaques may ulcerate and the turbulence in the blood flow allows the build up of clumps of platelets which eventually block the vessel. This process is not just happening in the coronary arteries, but any diminution of the blood flow here is likely to have the most dramatic consequences. The immediate result is *ischaemia*, or lack of blood flow to the organ supplied, in this case the *myocardium*, and this may be sudden and dramatic in the form of a heart attack, or gradual over the months or years as angina.

The early pathologists, who were a down-to-earth lot, called these deposits of cholesterol 'porridge', but they were also versed in the classics so they used the Greek term *atheroma*, and later *atherosclerosis* (which means 'hard porridge'). It is atherosclerosis which is responsible for a plethora of pathology in the form of strokes, gangrene of the feet and renal failure as well as myocardial ischaemia, depending on which vessels are most involved.

Who Develops Ischaemia?

Before the age of 50 myocardial ischaemia is predominantly a male disease, but after the menopause women gradually catch up until by the age of 60 the two sexes are about equal. Moreover the average age of onset is decreasing and some men are noticing symptoms in their thirties or even younger.

Diet plays a part, not only in the development of atherosclerosis, but also in the amount of work the heart has to perform in someone who is obese. It is generally considered, despite the rearguard action by the milk marketing board, that *saturated fats* in the form of dairy products and meat are largely responsible for the excessive amount of lipid and *cholesterol* in the blood, and recently it has been shown that a diet deficient in *linoleic acid*, present in fish and unsaturated oils, may lead to heart attacks.

Smoking approximately doubles the risk of ischaemic heart disease, for cigarette smokers have an increased quantity of atheroma. Moreover the nicotine present in the smoke narrows the arteries still further, and also inhibits the uptake of linoleic acid.

High blood pressure induces ischaemia because of the extra work which the muscles of the ventricles have to do, which requires a greater flow of blood, and an excess of salt predisposes to this.

Stress and competetive behaviour have an affect on the heart, although these are not easy to quantify. Physical activity is, of course, beneficial by improving the collateral circulation in those vessels which are not obstructed, and this in itself improves one's chances in the event of a heart attack. Psychologists have noticed that driving, ambitious individuals (labelled Type A) are at much greater risk than those called Type B who are able to take life as it comes.

Oral contraceptives, especially those which contain a high proportion of oestrogens, have recently been shown to increase the risk of coronary heart disease slightly.

Angina Pectoris

As the supply of blood and hence oxygen to the heart muscle declines, a form of cramp-like pain in the chest develops, known as *angina*. This is felt mostly at times of physical and emotional stress when the heart's demand for blood is highest, but anaemia may sometimes bring it on. The amount of exertion needed is similar with each attack, so the patient soon learns to anticipate where to ease up. Walking against a cold wind is especially provocative but heavy meals or smoking can also precipitate angina. One useful diagnostic sign is that angina comes on during, not after exercise, and is relieved by rest within a few minutes.

The *character* of the pain is typical and is felt as a dull, tight, constricting pain, occasionally an ache but never a sharp, stabbing pain. It may easily be mistaken for indigestion as the ache may be in the lower chest and even be accompanied by belching. The *distribution* of the pain varies, but is always the same in an individual and usually starts behind the sternum (*retrosternal pain*) but cannot accurately be located by pointing. It may radiate down the inside of the left or even occasionally the right arm to the hand, ending in the 4th and 5th fingers. In a few it may be felt in the jaw or the upper abdomen.

A particularly serious type of angina is that known as *unstable angina*, as this may herald a *heart attack*. It is recognised by an increase in the severity of the pain and a change in its radiation pattern. The pain may come on spontaneously and fluctuate for several days and then end or go on to become an attack, and it is patients who develop these symptoms who are usually offered surgery in the form of a bypass graft, using a vein removed from the leg in the hope that this will prevent an infarction (see below).

Heart Attack

When a heart attack occurs the pain usually starts at rest without warning, often during sleep, and is similar in distribution to angina but much more severe, sometimes causing *sweating, nausea, vomiting* and *extreme fear*. It lasts much longer than angina and may go on for several hours without stopping. In one third of cases the attack follows unstable angina, and in about one in ten (usually elderly) there is no pain at all but only sweating, dizziness and breathlessness. In general, the greater the amount of myocardial damage the more severe are the symptoms.

The cause of the attack is a sudden cessation in blood flow as the coronary artery supplying one of the ventricles, usually the left, becomes thrombosed with blood or platelets which collect on the ulcerated plaque. This denies the muscle any nutrition and it promptly dies, becoming filled with coagulated blood which turns dark red and comes to resemble a piece of salami, so has been endowed with the fanciful name of *infarction* (from the Latin infarcere = stuffing). This *myocardial infarction*, to give it the correct name, will then proceed to contract and eventually become a scar (assuming that the patient survives the assault) but until it has done so the heart and circulation are at some risk of certain complications which may ensue.

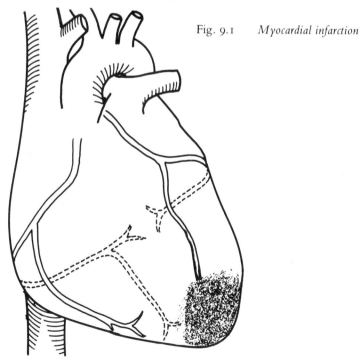

Fig. 9.1   *Myocardial infarction*

The complications depend to a large extent where the infarct occurred and how much tissue died. Obviously in the case of a massive infarction which follows a major blockage the chances of death are high, and this is the outcome in about 40% of cases, one third of whom will perish immediately.

If the person survives, however, the pumping power of the heart will be too feeble to maintain enough pressure to supply the tissues, when the person is said to be *shocked* and they will then be very cold, pale and clammy and may even be unconscious. Once recovered, the injured left ventricle may have difficulty expelling all the blood it receives, and some will get held up in the lungs causing *pulmonary oedema* and breathlessness, one of the early signs of *heart failure* (see below).

Even if the patient does not succumb to the immediate attack they are still not out of the wood, and another third die within the first 48 hours. The usual reason for this is the involvement of the conduction pathways of the heart in the infarction, so that an *arrythmia* or irregular rhythm occurs and the heart starts to beat in a wild or erratic fashion. These arrythmias are broadly speaking of two kinds, those involving the atria only and those involving the ventricles, and it is for this reason that patients are monitored with a cardiograph continuously in hospital. If the disruption is near the beginning of the conducting system, in the atria, then these will either beat very fast (*atrial flutter*) or irregularly (*atrial fibrillation*). The pulse will accordingly be rapid but regular at about 150/minute in the case of flutter, or totally irregular if there is atrial fibrillation.

However these atrial abnormalities are much less ominous than arrhythmias which arise in the ventricles. Here the impulse may be entirely blocked in its passage, so the heart beats very slowly at the rate set by the ventricles of about 40–50 a minute, known as *heart block*, and it is in situations like this that a temporary pacemaker may be required. Or new *ectopic beats* arise from a spontaneous source and these may become so rapid that they lead to *ventricular fibrillation* with the ventricles just quivering but unable to pump. Defibrillation can be attempted by applying an electric shock to the heart which temporarily stuns it and then usually allow normal rhythm to return.

As the wall of the ventricle heals it may on occasions bulge outwards to form a swelling known as an *aneurysm*

(Gr = dilation), and this will obviously impair the efficiency with which the heart pumps. If the infarction involves the inner lining of the heart, the endocardium, then this becomes roughened and attracts a clot of blood to stick to it called a *mural thrombus* which may later break off and enter the circulation as an *embolus* (Gr = wedge), ending up perhaps in the brain or leg to interfere with the blood supply there and possibly an infarction of those tissues. Finally the outer layer or pericardium may be involved and become inflamed leading to *pericarditis*. If this happens there is a recurrence of the pain a few days later, but this time a sharper, stabbing pain accompanied by a slight fever (the post-myocardial infarction syndrome).

Blood Pressure

The heart pumps blood around the body under pressure which varies according to the phase of the cardiac cycle, and this is felt at the wrist as a pulse wave. The highest pressure in the vessel coincides with the systolic phase of the ventricle and so is called the *systolic pressure*, while the trough of the wave occurs when the heart relaxes, the *diastolic pressure*. Even during diastole a flow is maintained in the arteries because of the elastic quality of their walls, so the diastolic pressure does not fall to zero and in fact reflects the state of the arterioles and their ability to relax.

Several factors influence our BP. The immediate one is the *contractile force of the heart*, so if the blood supply to the myocardium is defective it may be unable to contract forcefully and the BP drops suddenly to cause shock as we have already seen. Secondly the *volume of blood* which has to be pumped will influence the pressure, which also drops if we suddenly start to bleed heavily, but equally increases if our blood contains an excessive amount of salt, as the volume of fluid in the body is increased (because the kidneys are so efficient at retaining salt but have to retain an equal amount of water to dilute it). Thirdly the *peripheral resistance* of the arterioles can modify the BP considerably. This is done by constricting or dilating the muscular walls by a change in autonomic tone under the control of the vasomotor centre in the brain, which is in turn influenced by emotional factors such as anxiety, stress etc. All these factors serve to adjust our BP to the varying needs of the body at different times, but sometimes the mechanism malfunctions and high blood pressure or *hypertension* ensues and slowly damages certain organs.

Causes of Hypertension

If the kidneys become diseased then they respond by secreting large amounts of the hormone *renin* whose function is to constrict the arterial walls and so elevate the pressure in the vessels, and this is what happens in *nephritis, chronic pyelitis, polycystic kidneys* and probably to a degree in *toxaemia of pregnancy*. Certain hormonal abnormalities, such as an excess of cortisone in *Cushing's syndrome* or of oestrogens in the case of oral contraceptives in some who are susceptible will also bring about what is known as *secondary hypertension* but this is not, however, the usual cause of hypertension. About 90% of those with high blood pressure have *primary essential hypertension* which means that they have no demonstrable abnormality in any bodily system and the direct cause of their condition is unknown. Some will have a family history of 'blood pressure', some will be overweight but many are outwardly fit and healthy with no signs of anything amiss.

Consequences of Hypertension

Until the condition has been present for a good number of years and one of the target organs like the heart, brain or kidney is affected there are no symptoms apparent and the condition cannot be diagnosed unless someone takes the blood pressure (see below). Eventually the *left ventricle* of the heart enlarges or *hypertrophies* to produce the extra power required and this may be detectable clinically as a heaving impulse on the left border of the chest. By then the blood supply to the myocardium is often inadequate and the heart begins to fail, the patient experiencing breathlessness from the accumulating pulmonary oedema, and sometimes even sustaining a *myocardial infarction*. The other main organ affected is the brain, in which the increased pressure may lead to a *stroke* (see chapter 17) especially in the elderly in whom the vessels are somewhat hard and brittle.

A more sinister type of hypertension sometimes arises in younger people when the blood pressure rapidly accelerates to very high levels in the space of a few weeks and causes severe headaches and visual problems. This is known as *malignant hypertension* and is usually fatal within a few months unless promptly treated. Because the patient is young the heart is able to withstand the greatly elevated pressure, and the brunt of the attack falls on the kidneys which become congested and go into *renal failure*. There is a marked thickening in the inner layer of the larger renal arterioles which therefore fail to supply the glomeruli and these atrophy, a change which is mirrored in the retina and can be directly observed with the ophthalmoscope.

Taking Blood Pressure

This is done by wrapping a cuff around the upper arm and occluding the artery using an instrument called a *sphygmomano-meter* (Gr. sphingo = throttle, the Sphinx was a monster who throttled her victims). The pressure is then lowered until a soft, tapping sound is just heard caused by the turbulence of the blood in the narrowed artery, and this signifies the systolic pressure. As the cuff continues to deflate the distortion of the artery lessens and the turbulence becomes a smooth flow until eventually the sound disappears altogether, at the point where the normal contours of the artery have been regained. This represents the diastolic pressure and is sometimes heard as a muffling of the sound rather than its disappearance.

If problems arise it is probably because (a) the stethoscope has not been placed exactly over the brachial artery (or even has the hole occluded), (b) the elbow is bent or has a tight sleeve over it, (c) the arm is very fat which makes accuracy difficult, (d) the valve in the sphygmomanometer has not been unscrewed/screwed up or (e) you have not had enough practice! If a high reading is obtained then it should be checked when the practitioner and the patient have rested quietly for a few minutes.

Interpreting Blood Pressure

In Western societies, both the systolic and the diastolic pressure increase gradually with age and this is thought to be a reflection of the consumption of salt in our diet as it remains stable in 'low salt' communities. The maximal accepted values for the systolic pressure are generally regarded as the age of the patient plus 100, measured in mm of mercury, so the systolic pressure of a young person would be up to about 130 mm. As regards the diastolic pressure there is less agreement about the level at which the label 'abnormal' should be applied, but the graph in figure 9.2 gives an indication of average readings and it is well to be suspicious of levels of over 100.

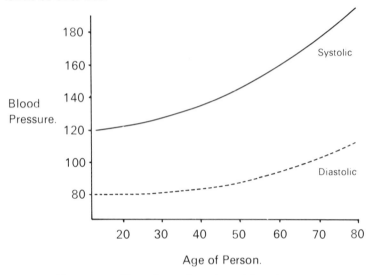

Fig. 9.2   *Upper limit of systolic and diastolic pressures*

Heart Failure

When the heart is unable to perform its primary function of pumping blood to the tissues it is said to have failed, but as the pump is a double one things are not quite so straightforward since the left ventricle ejects at a pressure of about 120 mm of Hg, whereas the right is only operating at a pressure of about 25 mm. Moreover, as we have seen, the left ventricle is much more frequently affected by ischaemic heart disease and hypertension, so it is this one which usually fails – *left ventricular failure* or *LVF*. Failure of a chamber of the heart has two consequences, firstly insufficient pressure is generated to perfuse the tissues ahead, sometimes called 'forward failure', but also excessive quantities of blood are held back and clog up the tissues behind (backward failure). So we can see that there are two groups of symptoms involved with each type of failure.

Left Ventricular Failure is usually the result of *ischaemia* or *hypertension*, less commonly *valvular disease* or *cardiomyopathy*. It is the natural consequence of old age in a heart which beats about 28 billion times in the average lifetime, so breathlessness (dyspnoea) on exertion comes to us all in time. This is because blood which cannot be pumped through the left ventricle congests the lung capillaries and prevents the rapid diffusion of oxygen, the pressure causing plasma to leak into the alveoli and cause the slight cough so common in the elderly.

While the person is up and about during the day, most of this congestion occurs at the base of the lungs and is not too much of a problem. However, after a few hours in bed, the slowing of the heart coupled with the redistribution of the fluid may cause him or her to wake gasping for breath with severe dyspnoea and a wet cough with pink, frothy sputum. This is known as *acute LVF* or *cardiac asthma* on account of the wheeze, which is caused by the airways filling with oedema fluid. Some relief is obtained by sitting forward (orthopnoea) so that the fluid drains back to the base of the lungs. In extreme situations there is faintness, sweating and cyanosis, and such cases are usually caused by an acute myocardial infarction.

Right Ventricular Failure. Sooner or later the congested capillaries of the lungs resulting from left ventricular failure will exert a back pressure on the right ventricle, and failure of the right side of the heart will follow. Or it sometimes happens that the right ventricle is affected by ischaemia or valvular disease and is unable to pump blood into the lungs. In this case the back pressure will be on blood in the peripheral veins, particularly those in the feet, and so the first sign is usually oedema of the ankles which start to swell (although swollen ankles also arise from other causes such as varicose veins). The jugular veins in the neck become visibly distended with a pulse that rises and falls with the heartbeat.

Many cases of right sided heart failure are not due to pathology in the heart at all, but occur because the circulation of blood through the lungs is impeded by lung diseases, especially chronic bronchitis and emphysema (see chapter 11). The pressure in the pulmonary circulation then rises in a manner similar to that which occurs in the systemic circulation in essential hypertension, causing the right ventricle to enlarge until it can no longer cope, when it fails. To this state of affairs the rather quaint phrase *cor pulmonale* has been given, meaning literally 'heart from the lungs', in other words heart disease secondary to lung disease.

Congestive Heart Failure. Although pure right or left sided heart failure does occur, it must be remembered that as both sides work together it is common for a degree of each to coexist and the term congestive heart failure is then used. The reason for this is that several conditions such as anaemia and thyrotoxicosis cause an increased demand for blood from both sides equally, so they fail together, and secondly because the kidney responds to a lack of perfusion by retaining salt and water, thus compounding the problem and causing the common symptom of peripheral oedema. It is for this reason that salt restriction is desirable, and why diuretics are usually used in orthodox treatment.

Pericarditis

This is an inflammatory condition of the pericardium, due to *infection, neoplasm, myocardial infarction* or sometimes *rheumatoid arthritis*. The usual cause is a virus, when it may follow a chest infection especially in young men. The pain is accompanied by a fever, and is felt as a sharp pain over the front of the chest, sometimes referred to the left shoulder as well. It is made worse by deep inspiration and lying down on the left side, and on listening carefully a soft creaking noise called a *friction rub* may be heard superimposed on the heartbeat. Pericarditis not uncommonly follows a few days after a myocardial infarction, and may also be a feature of a bronchial carcinoma which is extending directly towards the heart.

In certain cases fluid may collect within the pericardial sac, a *pericardial effusion*, and this may accumulate quite rapidly and compress the heart so that it cannot pump adequately and begins to fail. If there is a tubercular infection a very rigid and thickened pericardium may result, called *constrictive pericarditis*, and produce similar symptoms.

Rheumatic Fever

Fifty years ago the phrase 'acute rheumatism' was regarded as an ominous portent of heart disease to come and synonymous with what is now more often termed *rheumatic fever*. It is a condition which tends to affect children and adolescents, and although much less common now it is still a scourge of the developing world and responsible for most heart disease there. The decrease in this country started well before the advent of antibiotics and probably reflects changes in the virulence of the *haemolytic streptococcus*, the organism which is intimately related to the condition. For the fever is preceded 2–3 weeks before by an infection of the bacterium, usually in the throat, and this stimulates the production of antibodies by the lymph glands. Unfortunately these antibodies then go on to attack the connective tissues of the heart and joints, which by coincidence have a protein structure identical to that of part of the streptococcus.

The first symptoms of rheumatic fever are an abrupt *arthritis* which flits from one large joint to another every few days, accompanied by sweating and a rapid pulse. At the same time the heart is also being damaged in the process, leading to heart failure and breathlessness when the myocardium is involved, but also attacking the valves to give rise to small growths and irregularities on them. These interfere with the flow of blood through the heart and cause turbulence which is heard as a *heart murmur* and over the months, as the acute inflammation dies down, the valve becomes permanently deformed and fibrotic – *rheumatic heart disease*. The valve most frequently affected is the mitral valve, and also to a lesser extent the aortic, and these may either end up narrowed – *stenosis*, or leaking and unable to close properly – *incompetent*. The long-term consequences of this are that back pressure will congest the lungs and eventually even the right ventricle, so various operations have been devised for restructuring or replacing the affected valves.

The acute disease, which as the saying goes 'licks the joints but bites the heart', is not confined to these two organs alone, and lesions appear sometimes on the skin as the typical rash of *erythema marginatum*. This is an erythema, or reddening of the skin, in patches which have a distinct margin, so that they look a little like ringworm without the scaling. A more frequent feature are the *subcutaneous nodules* seen on the bony protuberances such as the elbows and knees. These are painless swellings under the skin such as are also seen in rheumatoid arthritis. Another distinctive feature sometimes seen is *Sydenham's chorea* (not to be confused with Huntington's chorea, an inherited disability). The word comes from the Greek 'chorus', which was the dance performed during a play, and describes the spontaneous writhing and twisting movements which take place for a few days. In their mild state they may not amount to much and be mistaken for fidgetting and restlessness, so many cases of rheumatic fever are only diagnosed retrospectively when the heart murmur is noticed or the patient becomes breathless.

Congenital Heart Disease

Not all heart murmurs are rheumatic in origin, however, and about 1 in 100 babies are born with a persistant heart murmur of whom a quarter have a defect serious enough to require surgery. The heart develops from a series of folds in the main blood vessel during the seventh week of embryonic life and minor irregularities easily occur, usually for no apparent reason but sometimes as a result of maternal infections such as rubella. The common abnormalities are either obstructions to the flow of blood or abnormal communications between the chambers – a 'hole in the heart'.

These latter defects are the most common variety and consist of defects in the septum between the left and right sides of the heart so are called ventricular septal defects (VSD) or atrial septal defects (ASD) accordingly. They range from minute pinhole-size apertures to holes large enough to *'shunt'* much of the blood across from the left to the right ventricle each time the heart beats, flooding the lungs with blood and causing cyanosis (the 'blue baby'). As the child gets older most of these holes tend to diminish in size, but some of the larger ones will need an operation to protect the lungs from future damage from pulmonary hypertension.

Stenosis or narrowing may also occur, principally to the pulmonary valve which may eventually cause the right side of the heart to fail, or to the aortic arch itself, when it is known as *'coarctation of the aorta'*. This is a narrowing of the aorta at any point along its course but usually the arch, and effectively prevents blood reaching the tissues beyond. The heart must therefore generate tremendous pressure in its attempt to push blood through and enlarges to a considerable size unless the obstruction is relieved. For this reason it is important to routinely examine the femoral pulse of all newborn babies as this will be missing in such cases.

Cardiomyopathy

During its lifetime the heart muscle gets through an enormous amount of work, and is therefore very susceptible to changes not only in its blood supply but also in its general nutrition. If there is a shortcoming in vitamins, thyroxine or other nutrients, as may occur particularly in alcoholism, the muscle will weaken, the heart dilate, and eventually failure will occur, a state known as *congestive cardiomyopathy*. Another type of cardiomyopathy is congenital in origin and stems from an inability of the cells to contract fully, so they eventually swell up and impede the flow of blood through the heart as *hypertrophic cardiomyopathy*. In both cases there is progressive weakness, dyspnoea and fatigue, with palpitations and irregularities of the heartbeat which may be dangerous.

10

Vessels: Disorders of Perfusion

Every part of the body with the exception of the epidermis and the cornea is supplied with blood by a huge network of vessels which stretch for a total of about 75,000 miles in all, enough to go round the world three times! The vast majority of this network is composed of the tiny capillaries, but the arteries with their elastic and muscular walls are critical for the regulation of the fluctuating pressure of the heart yet must not impede the smooth flow of blood. As was indicated in the last chapter, the impediment when it occurs is usually in the form of *atheroma*, of which there has been a sevenfold increase since the turn of the century. The onset of atheroma is particularly accelerated in hypertensives and smokers, and also in those who have excess cholesterol in the blood (*hypercholesterolaemia*) either of diabetic, hypothyroid or familial origin.

Atheroma is not the only condition to affect the arteries, however, and as we age deposits of calcium form in the medial coat and lead to 'hardening of the arteries'. To a large extent this is a natural process and does not cause any narrowing of the artery itself but may be felt as the cord-like arteries in elderly people.

The Aorta

This is the major vessel leaving the heart and as such must bear the brunt of the pressure exerted by the left ventricle. Syphilis was once a very significant source of damage to the aorta, as the elastic coat was attacked and lead to weakness and aneurysms in the ascending part. This gradually enlarged and compressed the structures of the mediastinum until its final dramatic rupture, sometimes into the trachea or oesophagus.

Aneurysms of the aorta still occur but of a different type; they affect the descending thoracic or abdominal aorta and cause it either to *bulge* or to *split* so that blood enters the medial coat and 'dissects' it for a short distance before either re-entering the lumen or rupturing through the outer wall leading to rapid death. Such *dissecting aneurysms* occur mainly in middle aged men and cause a severe, tearing pain in the chest and back, accompanied by shock, so they are often misdiagnosed as the more common myocardial infarction.

The other type of abdominal aneurysm, which bulges rather than splits, is due to atheromatous weakening of the whole wall and usually occurs in the abdominal aorta of older people, often without symptoms or with just vague lower back or abdominal pains. A swelling which pulsates will be felt in the abdomen, and this will often remain constant for many years, but will require surgery and a replacement graft if it starts to enlarge. If it occurs in the chest it may press on the trachea or oesophagus and cause a persistant cough or difficulty swallowing.

Intermittent Claudication

The word 'claudication' means to limp (the Roman emperor Claudius derived his name from this characteristic), and signifies the hallmark of the problem — an aching, cramp-like pain which occurs in the muscles of the calf or foot after walking a short distance, and which is alleviated by resting for a few minutes, only to return on further exertion. The cause is severe narrowing of the femoral or popliteal arteries, usually in men and almost always from atherosclerosis. The earliest symptoms are cramps in the calves at night, followed by coldness, blueness and loss of hair over the lower calf. The skin is dry to the touch as sweating is impaired, and when it is blanched by pressure takes a long time for the colour to be restored. The pulses will often be absent in the foot, knee or groin, depending on the site of the blockage, and eventually the ischaemia becomes so severe that the viability of the skin is affected and it may ulcerate and become gangrenous, requiring amputation.

Diabetics are prone to occlusion of particularly the smaller arterioles of the feet, especially if their diabetes has been badly controlled. Since they are also liable to skin infections, and may also have impairment of sensation, the combination not infrequently leads to surgery, so diabetics have to be scrupulous about the least injury to their feet lest they develop ulceration.

Raynaud's Disease

This is characterised by intermittent episodes of *pallor* and *cyanosis* of the digits, especially the fingers, usually precipitated by exposure to cold or by exercise. The small arteries react by constricting and the fingers turn white, then blue and finally bright red and begin to throb and tingle as the arteries dilate again. It is a genetic condition which affects younger women and may sometimes be so severe as to lead to ulceration of the fingertips. Some patients develop Raynaud's phenomenon as a result of pressure on the brachial artery from an extra cervical rib in the neck, or from using vibrating machinery, or as a side-effect of drugs such as beta-blockers, the contraceptive pill or ergot. Occasionally it may be the first symptom of a collagen disease such as systemic lupus erythematosis or scleroderma.

Chilblains are a more localised form of reaction to the cold and are usually seen on the hands or the feet as areas of swollen and itchy skin which turns red or purple. They may occur in those whose hands get repeatedly chilled and then warmed too quickly in front of a fire.

Temporal Arteritis

Although not common, it is very important not to overlook this condition, also known as *cranial* or *giant cell arteritis*, as the consequences may be serious. It is an inflammatory disorder of the arteries of the head, especially the temporal artery which can be felt just in front of the ear, but which becomes thickened and tender, causing headaches and great sensitivity of the scalp for reasons which are not clear but possibly have something to do with allergy. Nor is only the temporal artery involved, for other arteries may inflame and become blocked, particularly the ophthalmic artery supplying the eye which may lead to blindness unless urgently treated.

There is a close association between this disease and *polymyalgia rheumatica*, both occurring exclusively in the elderly and either coexisting or leading from one to the other. Polymyalgia is, as the name suggests, characterised by aching of the muscles particularly of the pelvis and shoulders, and there is often weight loss and a fever signifying a generalised disorder.

The Veins

These are more than just collecting channels, they form a reservoir which contains over half the blood in circulation, flowing gently under a low pressure. This predisposes them to thrombosis, especially when subjected to compression or stagnation, and because their walls are relatively thin, wherever back pressure occurs they are likely to dilate and form a varix or several *varices* (L = bubble). Varices occur most often in the legs, where gravity has the greatest affect, and also at the anal margin (*haemorrhoids*), the lower end of the oesophagus (*oesophageal varices*) and in the scrotum or labia (*varicocele*).

Varicose Veins

These are dilated, tortuous, superficial veins in the legs, either the *short saphenous vein* on the outer aspect or more commonly the *long saphenous vein* which runs from ankle to groin on the inner aspect (Gr. saphenous = outstanding). They are accompanied early on by cramps and itching, later by aching and heaviness particularly after standing and finally by such complications as ulceration and inflammation (*phlebitis*).

In most cases varicose veins arise because of an inherited defect of the valves of the legs, but the pressure from a pregnancy or occupations involving standing for long periods also predispose, as does damage to the valves from thrombophlebitis. Once a valve is damaged, the one below is subjected to an even greater strain and this will also fail until eventually the greatest pressure is exerted at the ankle. Here blood will leak out of the vessel and stain the skin, causing the irritation and dryness of *varicose eczema*, with eventual excoriation and infection. The skin may become devitalised and oedematous, finally breaking down as a *varicose ulcer* which may take many months to heal.

Although ulcers around the ankle are usually of varicose origin, they also arise in a number of other conditions, the main ones being *diabetes, intermittent claudication* and *rheumatoid arthritis.* African or West Indian patients with *sickle cell anaemia* are also prone to leg ulceration.

Apart from ulceration varicose veins may on occasions rupture and the resulting haemorrhage become a little alarming. It may be controlled by elevating the leg and compressing the vein with a finger until the bleeding ceases, then bandaging firmly with a crepe bandage. If a varicose vein becomes acutely red, tender and inflamed then the patient is probably developing phlebitis, or more accurately *thrombophlebitis* as the vein becomes thrombosed early on. Although painful, the condition is restricted to the superficial veins as a rule, and does not give rise to emboli which normally come from the deep veins of the calf. On occasions phlebitis may arise in other veins in the body such as the brachial vein in the axilla, either as a result of local trauma – e.g. using a crutch – or as part of a general condition called *thrombophlebitis migrans*. In this the phlebitis migrates to other areas of the body and causes a flitting, tender cord where the vein has clotted, and may be the first sign of an underlying cancer, especially in the pancreas.

Deep Vein Thrombosis (DVT)

This is a situation where the blood clots within one of the deep veins of the calf or pelvis, usually because the flow has become rather sluggish, the blood has become dehydrated or trauma has occurred in the area. Such events occur after abdominal surgery, heart attacks and childbirth, if the patient is confined to bed and there is a sluggish circulation. In other cases the cause is an increased tendency for the blood to clot, either because of abnormal proteins present in certain cancers or due to drugs such as oestrogens (present in only very small quantities in contraceptive pills now, but sometimes used to treat cancers of the prostate and breast).

The patient usually, but not always, experiences some aching in the calf which may swell slightly. They may also be a little feverish and feel unwell. However in many cases there are no symptoms and the diagnosis is not made until complications set in. The main sequel to a deep venous thrombosis is that a piece breaks off and travels as an embolus up the inferior vena cava to the right side of the heart and thence to the lungs where it blocks the arteriole in which it comes to rest, causing ischaemia and possibly infarction. A *pulmonary embolus* is one of the main causes of sudden death after an operation, if it is large enough to obstruct a major artery, and is often immediately preceded by a desire to empty the bowels because of the stimulation of the vagus nerve as the embolus traverses the inferior vena cava, hence many of these patients are found collapsed in the toilet (one reason why hospital toilets have no locks!).

If an *infarction* of the lung occurs there will be a sharp *pleuritic pain* and some *difficulty breathing*, sometimes followed by a slight *haemoptysis* a while later. Occasionally the DVT itself is symptomless and there are merely recurrent episodes of dyspnoea, wheeze and faintness until the patient develops pulmonary hypertension as the pulmonary tree is progressively blocked by emboli.

11

Lungs: Disorders of Breathing

Our lungs are in constant contact with the air, so much so that they might almost be thought of as being outside the body, yet they are extremely delicate organs and rely for their protection on the mechanisms of the upper part of the respiratory tract where the air is warmed, humidified and purified. It is therefore this area which is likely to become damaged by pollution or infected by bacteria and viruses to cause what are known as *upper respiratory tract infections* or URTIs and in turn this may lead to catarrh. The reaction of any mucus membrane to stimulation is to exude mucus to protect itself, unfortunately the nasal passages are somewhat tortuous and narrow and may contain obstructions such as polyps and this prevents the free drainage of the catarrh which remains to cause a stuffy nose, sinusitis, earache or a chronic cough.

Upper Respiratory Tract Infections

The common cold (coryza) is a pattern of symptoms associated with numerous different viruses, and featuring nasal obstruction and discharge, sore throat and a cough which last about 7–10 days. The mucus is clear to begin with but then becomes yellow or green with bacterial infection by about the third day. Children are especially susceptible during the first few years of life and again when they start school. The main complications are otitis media in children, sinusitis in adults and hypostatic broncho-pneumonia in the elderly or bedfast.

Laryngitis may be an accompaniment to a cold or may occur alone, especially in children, when it appears as *croup*. Adults developing laryngitis may lose their voice (aphonia) or complain of hoarseness, and usually recover within a day or two. Chronic hoarseness is likely to be due to inflammation of the chords from smoking, overuse of the voice or allergy. Occasionally it may be from swelling of the vocal cords which occurs in myxoedema, or from a tumour or nodule. On occasions the throat has the sensation of a lump in the region of the larynx although no swelling is palpable, and this is often the result of unexpressed grief being choked back and may go under the name of a *globus hystericus*.

Sinusitis is a condition mainly of adults and teenagers, as childrens' sinuses do not develop fully until puberty. Acute sinusitis follows either a blockage of the opening by a cold or allergy, or from diving. There is pain and tenderness over the sinus involved, either above the eyes in frontal sinusitis or beside the nostrils and in the upper teeth, which feel long, in maxillary sinusitis. The sphenoid and ethmoid sinuses are further back and give less trouble. Chronic sinusitis may follow a physical obstruction such as a *deviated septum* or *polyp* which prevent free drainage, and these polyps are seen mostly in those with allergic rhinitis. The sinus fills with fluid and causes a postnasal drip with chronic catarrh and a persistant cough, and the fluid level within it may be seen by transilluminating the sinus through the mouth in a dark room using a bright torch.

Tonsillitis is often attributable to bacteria, especially strepto-cocci, but some cases involve viruses, either an adenovirus infection or glandular fever. The onset is sudden, with sore throat, fever, swollen tonsillar glands and malaise. The tonsils themselves are swollen and red, with pus or exudate visible in the crypts, and may go on to form an abscess known as a *quinsy* (peritonsillar abscess). Prior to the last war such symptoms were always a grave source of concern as they frequently indicated diphtheria, but this disease with its thick, white membrane adherent to the tonsils and toxic effect on the heart and nervous system is an extreme rarity nowadays.

Epiglottitis is a condition which is not common though serious when it appears, and is usually found in small children. It may initially be mistaken for croup, but the child is more severely ill and develops *stridor*, or noisy breathing, due to the obstruction of the swollen epiglottis which blocks the larynx. A particular strain of the bacterium Haemophilus influenzae is the usual cause.

Epistaxes or nose-bleeds are usually traumatic or spontaneous in origin and generally arise from the front of the nose on the septum, where they can be controlled by firm pressure between finger and thumb for at least five minutes continuously. Occasionally they are due to hypertension or even very rarely a bleeding disorder such as leukaemia or thrombocytopaenia. If they cannot be halted by pressure then the patient may need to have the nose packed with ribbon gauze.

Fig. 11.1   *Tonsillitis*

Acute Lung Infections

These normally follow the downward spread of a URTI into the lungs or the irritation of the trachea and bronchi by dust or chemicals, damp or cold. *Tracheitis* is a sore, scratchy retrosternal pain with only a little sputum unless it extends down into the bronchi as *acute bronchitis*, when there will be some wheeze with thick, yellow sputum and occasionally slight haemoptysis (coughing blood). The main risk is to babies, in whom the extension of the infection into the smaller bronchi, sometimes called *bronchiolitis*, has consequences similar to pneumonia and is one possible cause of cot death.

Influenza is a viral infection which gains its name from the fact that it was once thought to be under the influence of the stars which explained its periodic outbreaks as worldwide pandemics in which large numbers died of influenzal pneumonia. The most dramatic of these was the outbreak of 1918 when 20 million are said to have died, and more recently minor ones spread from Asia in 1957 and Hong Kong in 1968. There are three types of influenza virus, named A, B and C, of which only the first involves serious illness. However type A is able to mutate and replace itself with a new 'subtype' every few years and this may infect birds as well as humans, which carry it far and wide. The symptoms of 'flu are well known and usually transient unless the person is elderly or chronically ill when a type of viral pneumonia (see below) may develop and be rapidly fatal.

Pneumonia

Acute lobar pneumonia, sometimes called *pneumococcal pneumonia* after the organism involved, is seen less often now but classically occurs in previously healthy young adults who suddenly contract it after being chilled. They develop a high fever with a flushed, dry skin and uncontrollable shivering (rigors), sometimes with a herpes lesion on the mouth. There is aching and malaise followed by a cough with viscid sputum and later a little rust-coloured haemoptysis and even cyanosis. Respiration is rapid and shallow and often painful as the pleura is usually involved and leads to sharp, stabbing pains on breathing. In the untreated case the symptoms increase until they reach a 'crisis phase' at the end of a week or so, when they either make a dramatic recovery or die. One or more lobes of the lung are affected by the pneumococcus, and there is congestion and *consolidation* of the tissue, and sometimes spread of the organism throughout the body as septicaemia. If recovery is incomplete a *lung abscess* may remain in the lobe, or fluid may leak into the pleural space and cause a *pleural effusion*.

Atypical pneumonia is the name given to the more commonly met condition of today, as the symptoms come on more slowly and are more variable depending on which of the different organisms is involved. These are either viruses, chlamydia (such as those caught from birds in psittacosis), mycoplasma or the Legionella bacillus of *Legionnaire's disease*.

Although most are less virulent than lobar pneumonia, some, including Legionnaire's disease, have a significant mortality, and are more widespread than has been hitherto realised. The latter is a disease of especially the elderly and is more than just a pneumonia, involving the nervous system and digestive tract to cause confusion, hallucinations and diarrhoea.

Another form of infection of the lungs, occurring especially in the elderly and the debilitated, is **bronchopneumonia**. This may be due to a variety of organisms which are able to invade because of the lowered resistance of the body and the poor circulation through the lungs. The base of the lungs and the bronchi become slowly infected and collapse, leading to stupor, confusion and eventually peaceful death, so bronchopneumonia is often seen as the terminal event of many chronic diseases. It may be a sequel to such things as heart failure, cancer or chronic bronchitis, and a similar form of pneumonia is seen after the aspiration of vomit through epilepsy, alcohol or drug abuse.

Chronic Lung Infections

Any health worker in the industrial cities of the Midlands and North of England will have encountered **chronic bronchitis** or the 'English disease' as it is known. Although less common since the Clean Air Act of 1956, it still accounts for 30–40,000 deaths per annum with many more of its victims 'respiratory cripples', bound to their homes if not their beds by extreme breathlessness. Air pollution, dust, cigarette smoke and social factors combine to cause repeated attacks of acute bronchitis, especially in men, during the course of which the cilia are damaged so that eventually they cease to evacuate the debris which builds up and leads to a permanent irritation of the mucosal cells. These swell and pour out mucus which is coughed up each morning – the smoker's waking cough – and periodically become infected, causing still further damage and narrowing of the bronchioles. This leads to wheezing and sometimes to *emphysema*, the destruction of the partition walls of the alveoli and hence loss of the surface area of the lungs across which oxygen and carbon dioxide are transferred.

Either the bronchitis with its cough, wheeze and occasional haemoptysis, or else emphysema with its breathlessness is eventually likely to predominate in different individuals, and one of two clinical pictures will emerge. In the bronchitic the carbon dioxide cannot escape (it is more difficult to exhale than to inhale completely) and so is retained in the blood and causes central cyanosis which leads to drowsiness and a characteristic sluggish, Pickwickian appearance named the 'blue bloater'. The bloatedness is due in part at least to the oedema of the tissues which results from a degree of cor pulmonale (q.v.) common in this syndrome.

If **emphysema** predominates then ventilation (the movement of gas to and from the alveoli) is not a problem, but in order to transfer sufficient oxygen across his reduced alveolar area the patient must breathe more rapidly, and puffs rather than wheezes, usually blowing out his cheeks and holding his chest overinflated like a barrel. Cyanosis is not usually a problem because carbon dioxide can diffuse much more quickly than oxygen and readily escape, so they remain a healthy pink colour and are consequently known as 'pink puffers', but are usually extremely thin perhaps owing to the amount of energy expended on breathing. Some cases of emphysema are familial and are caused by a deficiency of the enzyme antitrypsin which normally plays a protective role, but this is probably only relevant in those who smoke.

Fig. 11.2   A. *Chronic bronchitis* and B. *Emphysema*

Bronchiectasis, like emphysema, is a destruction of tissue, but in this case involves the walls of the bronchi which dilate (Gr. ectasis = spread out). The pathological change which precedes and causes bronchiectasis is the occlusion of the small bronchi by secretions, coming from such diseases as *whooping cough, pneumonia* and *TB* especially during childhood. The lung tissue beyond the blockage collapses and the air is absorbed, a condition called *atalectasis* (Gr. atalos = delicate), and this shrinkage causes traction on the delicate walls of the infected bronchi which never regain their original shape but remain as dilated reservoirs of infection in different parts of the lung.

Thus arises the typical symptoms of cough with *profuse purulent sputum* and commonly *haemoptysis,* with loud rattling *crepitations* in the chest and eventually clubbing of the fingers (see below). Each morning at least the patient will require postural drainage by having someone assist loosen the sputum by smartly drubbing him on the back, when large quantities of often foul sputum will be coughed up. Sometimes the frontal sinuses are also chronically infected in this condition.

Fig. 11.3   *Bronchiectasis*

Cystic fibrosis gives rise to symptoms in children somewhat similar to those of bronchiectasis, but is a congenital disorder of the mucus produced in the glands of the pancreas and the bronchi. Owing to an enzyme defect this results in the mucus being much thicker than normal (hence the alternative name of *'mucoviscidosis'*), which leads to blockage of both the bronchioles and the pancreatic duct with both pulmonary and digestive consequences. The physical signs and symptoms in the chest are mainly those of cough and breathlessness but with the addition of wheezing and weight loss, and usually start at an early age. Cystic fibrosis is the commonest congenital condition in the West and occurs in about 1 in 2000 births, but may vary in severity and the mildest cases remain undiagnosed as asthma or just 'chestiness' in a growing child. The diagnosis is established by measuring the concentration of salt in the sweat which is always raised, but as yet no test is available to discern carriers of the gene. In a badly affected child there are frequent severe chest infections and only half will live beyond the age of 20.

Tuberculosis

Until recently the word itself was sufficient to alarm a whole generation who had experienced relatives struck down apparently indiscriminately by 'phthisis' or 'consumption' as it was known, and who were raised on the works of Hardy and Dickens with their dramatic descriptions of the inexorable progression of the disease. In fact TB was always a byproduct of the industrial revolution, affecting predominantly the young, the female and the poor, lurking especially in the damp alleyways of conurbations and the misty glens of the Western Isles. Today in this country TB is uncommon and usually seen in older men, often immigrants from the third world, and the once familiar sight of the mobile Xray unit is no longer seen. Periodically outbreaks still occur, however, and often when least expected, so one must be suspicious of the persistant cough, the night sweats and the unexplained loss of weight which are the usual presenting features.

The bacillus involved in this condition, *Mycobacterium tuberculosis*, has a unique mode of action which leads to the peculiar characteristics of the disease and its pathology. Its usual port of entry is via droplet infection into the lungs, but on occasions it may be swallowed and arrive in the wall of the gut, most often from infected milk. Once inside the body it is ingested by the large *macrophages*, which are monocytes that have migrated out of the blood to the tissues, but although these can ingest the bacteria they cannot kill them so a stalemate arises with nodules or 'tubercles' (L. =lump) arising at the site of entry – usually the lymph nodes of the hilum of the lung. These primary foci of infection become a battleground between the multiplying bacteria and their surrounding macrophages, and in their centre an area of debris or *caseation* (L. caseus = cheese) builds up. In most reasonably healthy inividuals the bacilli are destroyed eventually and the caseous area gradually calcifies to leave a 'shadow' on the lung and a positive reaction to the tuberculin or *Mantoux* (Heaf) test (which consists of challenging the body by inoculation with antigens from the protein wall of the bacillus and seeing whether it reacts). Thus ends the *primary infection*, usually acquired in childhood and usually without any symptoms apart from a slight cough and febrile illness, certainly nothing to make one suspect a potentially lethal disease.

However, in those whose immune system is defective in some way on account of chronic diseases such as diabetes, drug dependency or even simply lack of food, there develops a *progressive primary infection* as the organism overwhelms the inadequate macrophage response, and moves into the blood stream to set up metastatic foci elsewhere in the body, particularly the bones, kidneys, joints, skin, pericardium or adrenals. If the caseating focus is near a large vessel and invades it, then so-called *miliary tuberculosis* may spread seedling tubercles (L. milia = millet) to all areas of the body, including the brain and meninges, a frequently fatal outcome. On rare occasions the lymphatic glands in the neck become swollen with tubercular pus, and may discharge a cheesy material – the *scrofula* or 'King's evil' because it was reputably alleviated by the Royal touch!

More usual than a progressive primary infection is what is known as a *postprimary infection*, which occurs many years after the initial primary infection because the bacillus breaks out of the area and escapes control. This tends to be the type of case seen nowadays in older men, who reactivate an old focus and present with the typical symptoms of cough with haemoptysis, dyspnoea, fever with night sweats and loss of weight. The characteristic quality of the postprimary type of infection is that it tends to form large *cavities* in the lungs, particularly in the apex, and this is where the physical signs are often heard and what gives rise to the name of 'consumption'.

Children who have not been exposed to a primary infection, shown by a negative Mantoux or Heaf test, are theoretically at risk if in contact with an active case of TB. They may be offered immunisation with an attenuated form of the bacillus called BCG (Bacillus Calmette-Guerin).

Sarcoidosis

This is a somewhat mysterious disease, involving as it does so many different organs but with the lungs almost always playing a leading role. For many years it was thought to be a variety of TB as it is histologically very similar, but neither organisms nor caseation have ever been seen. The hallmark of the disease is the *granuloma*, a collection of chronic inflammatory cells, macrophages in particular. The name arises from the fact that granulomas were originally thought to be tumours with a granular appearance, and they are common to many other chronic diseases, such as TB, syphilis and leprosy.

A typical acute case starts in a young adult, with fever, stiff joints (especially the knees and ankles), swollen glands and breathlessness with a slight cough. A chest Xray will reveal that the mediastinal glands are enlarged and there is a diffuse mottling in the lungs where the granulomas are seen. The severity of the condition varies, but almost all cases resolve in 2–3 years without treatment, although steroids are given if more serious features are evident. These include involvement of the eyes (uveitis), the heart (cardiomyopathy) and the nervous system (nerve palsies and meningitis).

A common and inexplicable feature in the earlier stages of many cases is a tender, dark red discoloration of the calves known as *erythema nodosum*, looking rather like a series of bruises running down the shins. This skin disorder occurs as a result of other conditions as well, in particular streptococcal throat infections, rheumatic fever, TB and reactions to some drugs. It is a peculiar and significant symptom and if seen should be investigated further.

Bronchial Asthma

Asthma is one of the the most significant disorders of the lungs seen by practitioners today, as it is so common (occurring in about 1 person in 10 to some degree) and is responsible for over 2000 deaths annually. It is defined as a reversible (as compared to chronic bronchitis) narrowing of the bronchioles of the lung. Broadly speaking there are two main types of asthma, extrinsic and intrinsic, and several subsidiary ones such as exercise-induced asthma and occupational asthma due to inhaled chemicals and dust.

Atopic or **extrinsic asthma** is the common type occurring in children, especially boys, who have inherited an atopic (see chapter 2) response to various allergens such as pollen, animal fur and the house-dust mite found in bedding, dust etc. These children will usually be positive to skin tests for these allergens, and may exhibit other allergic tendencies such as hay fever, eczema or rhinitis, as will many of their relatives. It seems that these children inherit the liability to produce excessive quantities of antibodies in the form of immunoglobulins which renders them hypersensitive, so that the cells of the bronchioles react to the allergen violently and discharge chemicals such as histamine which make them constrict and swell up, so narrowing the airway. This leads to the characteristic wheeze and prolonged, difficult exhalation seen in an attack, which may come on quite suddenly. The exhalation is prolonged because it is essentialy a passive act accomplished by the elastic qualities of the lung, and this results in air becoming trapped in the overinflated chest giving it a barrel-shaped symmetry and limiting movement of the ribs, seen in severe chronic asthmatics.

The small bronchioles also produce mucus which eventually dries and plugs the air passages in a prolonged episode, leading to oxygen lack and cyanosis in a severe case. Most episodes of asthma occur at night and last 1–2 hours unless they are due to emotional causes or follow URTIs in which case they may be prolonged. In the event of an attack continuing for more than 6–8 hours the term 'status asthmaticus' is applied, and the risks are correspondingly increased. Between attacks the child may scarcely wheeze at all, but often has a characteristic *dry cough*, and this is usually the first sign of the onset of asthma.

Intrinsic asthma is the name given to that variety of asthma which emerges in later life and in which allergic stimuli play only a minor part. It is mostly seen in women in whom attacks of asthma occur against a background of general wheeziness, and it is in this group that most fatalities occur. There is a high incidence of nasal polypi in such people which complicates breathing still further, and they are sometimes allergic to aspirin which is liable to provoke a severe attack.

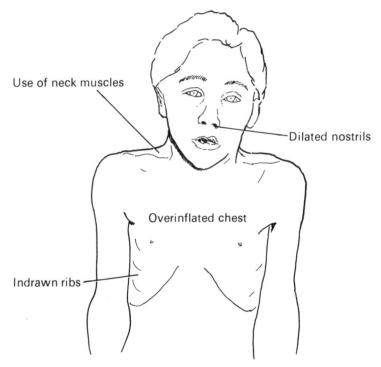

Fig. 11.4   *Atopic child with asthma*

Lung Cancer

Bronchial carcinoma, arising from the cells lining the small bronchi, is by far the commonest cause of cancer among men and has increased thirtyfold since the beginning of the century and is now responsible for about one death in every 20, although it is at last levelling off. Although women are much less likely to contract it, current smoking patterns among girls indicate that it will have overtaken breast cancer to reach the number one spot within the next few years. Because our bronchial mucosa is continually in contact with the environment it acts as a kind of 'pollution meter' for such substances as tars, soot, hydrocarbons and many other carcinogens, which means that the inhalation of others' tobacco smoke also increases our risk substantially. Depending on the amount smoked and the number of years of exposure, mutations of the cells result which eventually lead to malignant change.

The type of cancer and its rate of growth depends on its similarity to its parent cell, in other words the degree to which it has specialised or *differentiated* from a primitive cell. A cancerous cell which is a very crude imitation of its original tissue, i.e. is *undifferentiated*, tends to have few controls over its growth and is therefore highly malignant. Such cancers make up about half the cases and are sometimes termed 'oat-cell' carcinomas after their resemblance to an ear of the grain on the stalk.

Between the inception of a cancer and the appearance of symptoms lies a period of 2–3 years, during which time the tumour is growing locally, but at some point vessels and lymphatics are likely to be invaded and convey the malignant cells to a distant site in the form of a *metastasis*. The first evidence of anything amiss may therefore be from a symptom far removed from the area, such as an epileptic fit or a fracture, for lung cancer tends to spread to the *brain, bones, liver* and *adrenal glands*. Very often the first metastasis appears in the lymphatic tissues as a swollen lymph gland in the mediastinum first seen on Xray.

A 'typical' case of bronchial carcinoma would be a middle-aged man who smokes and gradually loses weight and feels unwell over a period of about six weeks, experiences a persistant and irritating cough and becomes a little breathless. Eventually he might experience some dull pain in the chest and cough up a little blood. When the tumour has enlarged enough to block the bronchus completely the lung beyond it will collapse (*atelectasis*) and become infected, leading to a fever and sudden worsening of symptoms. Later one of a number of different signs may appear, especially:

—*pleural effusion*. If the tumour lies in the outer part of the lung then its spread will take it to the pleura which reacts by secreting bloodstained fluid into the pleural cavity. This is always painful and accounts for much of the pain felt by patients with this disease, moreover the effusion may become infected and form an *empyema*, a collection of pus in the pleural cavity (this occasionally occurs after pneumonia also). Further, the pericardium itself may be invaded and lead to pericarditis.

—*superior vena cava syndrome* occurs when the enlarging growth compresses the thin-walled superior vena cava in the mediastinum and obstructs the blood returning to the heart, causing swelling and plethora of the neck and shoulders.

—*Horner's syndrome* (see chapter 19).

—*clubbing of the fingers*, a strange and inexplicable condition of the fingernails and to a lesser extent the toes, whereby the nails become increasingly curved and eventually swell like a drumstick. It is found in lung disorders such as TB, bronchiectasis, emphysema and alveolitis, in congenital heart disease and in cirrhosis, Crohn's disease and ulcerative colitis.

—*hoarseness* due to damage to the recurrent laryngeal nerve.

Respiratory Failure

Just as heart failure is the inability to pump blood, so respiratory failure is the inability to oxygenate it, and this may happen for two reasons. Firstly because the *ventilation* of the lungs, that is the movement of air in and out, is inadequate because of obstruction in some form or another – '*obstructive airways disease*', and this applies to any disorder where the bronchi are narrowed. But a second problem may also occur, that of *diffusion* across the alveolar membrane, and this is reduced when the membrane is thickened for any reason.

When ventilation is diminished, as happens in asthma and chronic bronchitis, the oxygen is unable to enter and the patient exhibits symptoms of *hypoxia* – confusion, dizziness, drowsiness and weakness, similar to those seen in altitude sickness where the oxygen content of the air is very low. This is the first indication that they are developing a dangerous state and require oxygen quickly. At the same time CO2 is retained in the alveoli as it cannot escape, and will eventually build up in the blood leading to a bluish tinge – '*central cyanosis*'. By the time this has happened there will be quite a severe degree of obstruction to the airways and treatment is urgent. Of course the distinction must be made between central cyanosis due to respiratory failure and peripheral cyanosis due to sluggishness of the blood in the periphery such as occurs on the lips and skin of those who are thoroughly chilled.

Impairment of diffusion of gas across the alveolar membrane is usually limited to oxygen alone, as CO_2 can move across much

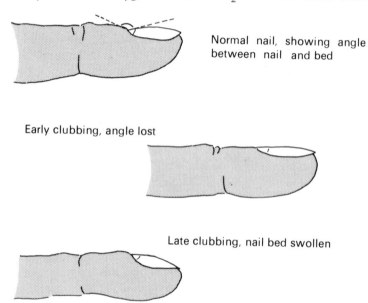

Normal nail, showing angle between nail and bed

Early clubbing, angle lost

Late clubbing, nail bed swollen

Fig. 11.5 *Normal nail, early and advanced clubbing*

more easily and quickly. Therefore cyanosis seldom appears in those who suffer from disease of their alveoli, and they are breathless without being cyanosed. As well as the destruction of the alveoli in emphysema already mentioned, a similar situation arises due to thickening of the membrane, either from fibrosis or inflammation from allergy – 'allergic alveolitis'. The latter condition is a result of inhaling moulds as in farmer's lung (hay), bird fancier's lung (bird droppings) etc. Pulmonary fibrosis occurs in connective tissue diseases such as rheumatoid arthritis, systemic lupus erythematosis and sarcoidosis, as well as in industrial lung disease caused by the inhalation of particles and chemicals. These particles generate a reaction in the alveoli and cause them to atrophy and thicken as tiny scars, leading to gross dyspnoea and clubbing of the fingers but no cyanosis. The main problem is that the fibrosis also extends to involve the lung capillaries and leads to great strain on the right ventricle which eventually fails from cor pulmonale.

The Pleura

These membranes surrounding the lungs contain a large number of pain receptors and their stimulation provokes a typically sharp, stabbing pain which is exacerbated especially by deep breathing. Because the pleura also cover the diaphragm which is innervated by the phrenic nerve, stimulation of this area may be felt as a pain referred to the shoulder.

Pleurisy is an acutely painful condition of the pleura which is normally the result of an acute infection of the underlying lung such as pneumonia, TB or some other lung condition. The most common non-infective causes are pulmonary embolus, a spreading carcinoma of the bronchus or occasionally rheumatoid arthritis. As well as giving rise to pains, the pleural membrane reacts by secreting fibrin which roughens the surface and may cause a *pleural rub* with each inspiration, audible with a stethoscope and not unlike a hinge which needs oiling. In some cases quantities of clear fluid are poured into the pleural space as a *pleural effusion*, and the lung is slowly compressed. If the fluid later becomes infected it changes to pus and an *empyema* is said to have occurred.

One specific cause of pleuritic-type pain is an infection by the Coxsackie B virus known as *Bornholm disease* after the island on which the first known outbreak occurred. Although the pain is pleuritic in character it is actually the underlying muscles of the chest wall which are mostly involved, hence the alternative name of 'epidemic myalgia'. The first symptoms are a fever and sore throat, followed a day or two later by the pains which may linger on for a week or more but will eventually clear without complications.

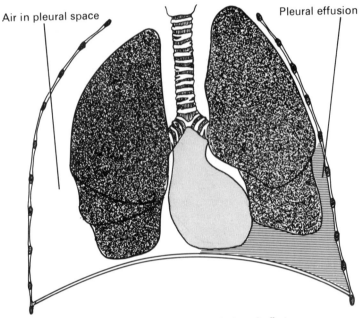

Air in pleural space

Pleural effusion

Fig. 11.6   *Pneumothorax and pleural effusion*

Pneumothorax is another condition involving the pleura and is caused by the rupture of a weak area of the outer wall of the lung, usually at the apex, which allows air to pass through into the thoracic cavity – the pneumothorax. The weakness is sometimes the result of chronic obstructive airways disease or emphysema, but may occur spontaneously in young adults, especially men who tend to be tall and thin. They experience a sudden pain in the side of the chest, perhaps while straining at something, followed by breathlessness as the lungs are compressed by the escaping air, but this often diminishes within half an hour or so as the other lung takes over and may even resolve spontaneously. If necessary the air can be drained out of the thorax via a one-way valve, when the pleura usually heals itself. However, spontaneous pneumothorax is likely to recur periodically and sometimes eventually requires an operation to seal the potential holes.

12

Mouth and Stomach: Disorders of Digestion

The mouth sustains a complex population of bacteria which maintains a stable ecology and under normal circumstances prevents pathogenic organisms from invading. On occasions, however, a mild alteration of the balance is responsible for furring of the tongue or halitosis (bad breath), but a more severe infection may occur after the resident population has been decimated by antibiotics, especially the broad-spectrum ones like tetracyclene, or else the normal function of the immune system impaired by drugs such as cortisone or diseases such as leukaemia, aplastic anaemia or AIDS. The resulting inflammation of the mouth is known as *stomatitis*, or *glossitis* if the tongue is predominantly involved. Inflammation of the lip is called a *cheilitis* or *cheilosis*.

Candida (monilia, thrush) is a common type of stomatitis, so-called because of its resemblance to the speckled appearance of a thrush's breast, and is seen on the cheek, tongue and palate of babies and the elderly or debilitated. Babies may contract the condition from the mother during birth, while the elderly sometimes develop chronic fissures at the corners of the mouth – 'angular cheilitis'. The surrounding area is red and sore, and the deposit cannot be scraped off, which distinguishes it from milk. Sometimes the oesophagus is involved and dysphagia may develop after a course of antibiotics.

Candida in the gut may be regarded as an indicator that the immune system is failing to some degree, as the organism is unable to colonise healthy tissue but invades when antibiotics, diabetes, corticosteroid therapy or immune defects such as AIDS or cancers prevail. The organism is particularly partial to sugar and other refined carbohydrates present in the diet of some, and is thought to be responsible for a variety of symptoms ranging from headaches and depression to cystitis and dyspepsia.

Ulcerating stomatitis may be caused by *herpes simplex* or by *aphthous ulceration* (Gr. apto = set on fire), when usually the tongue or inside of the cheek or lip is involved. Aphthae occur in crops as shallow, painful ulcers with a white rim and last for several days, appearing in those who are generally below par or suffer from food sensitivity or ulcerative colitis. Herpes simplex is a virus of the herpes family (qv) and attacks either the mouth and lips (HS1 or herpes labialis) or the genitalia (HS2 or herpes genitalis), producing a blister which rapidly ulcerates and crusts over. The first attack occurs in childhood in most people, and may involve a wide area of the gums and mouth – *herpetic stomatitis* – so the child is quite ill and feverish. Subsequent attacks, when the virus re-emerges from its dormant state, occur during periods of stress or exposure to the sun and wind and usually involve the lips (cold sore).

Leukoplakia is a chronic, premalignant condition involving the side of the tongue or the inside of the cheek, and appears as a thickened white plaque of tissue often at the site of continuous abrasion by such things as badly fitting dentures or a pipe. Most cases will eventually go on to become cancerous after a number of months or years, so should not be ignored.

Most cases of glossitis are due to a deficiency of *iron* or one of the *B vitamins*, especially B2 (Riboflavin), B12 or nicotinic acid. The moist velvety appearance is lost and the tongue appears smooth, sore and red or purple with atrophy of the papillae. The 'geographical tongue' is so-called because the loss of papillae is partial, leading to the resemblance to a map, but has no pathological significance. Heavy furring of the tongue may result from smoking or dietary disorders, and an extreme case is the 'black hairy tongue' which may relate to previous antibiotics. The 'strawberry tongue' of scarlet fever is described in chapter 3.

Gingivitis, or periodontitis as it is called when an area immediately surrounding the teeth is involved, is usually a result of poor dental hygiene. Organisms, especially Vincent's spir-ochaete, invade the tissue and cause leakage of pus (*pyorrhoea*) and even ulceration if neglected. Swelling of the gums may be a side-effect of phenytoin (Epanutin) therapy for epilepsy, and very rarely gum disease is due to vitamin C deficiency or scurvy.

The salivary glands seldom cause trouble unless there is much sepsis in the mouth, when the parotid particularly may inflame to cause a parotitis with a red, tender swelling. *Mumps* is a mild form of parotitis. In some cases of Parkinsonism there is an increase in salivation from the glands which may be troublesome, while in middle-aged women in particular the opposite may happen and the secretions from the salivary glands dry up, a condition known as *Sjogren's syndrome* and associated with drying of the joints and arthritis, sometimes also with absence of tears and gritty eyes. Another reason why one salivary gland may swell intermittently is the presence of a stone in the duct preventing the exit of saliva. The symptom will manifest mostly during meal times, and a *calculus* may be felt in the duct.

The Oesophagus

The only function of the oesophagus is to transport food through the thorax to the stomach, and as it is the narrowest part of the alimentary canal we can see why the main symptom of disease here is difficulty swallowing (*dysphagia*).

A *pharyngeal pouch* or diverticulum may appear in middle-age at the junction of the pharynx and the oesophagus where there is an area of potential weakness, and the patient will develop regurgitation of food. A swelling in the neck may be visible which will empty noisily under pressure, and eventually there will be some dysphagia at the top of the oesophagus. This is in contrast to that sometimes felt at the lower end in those who develop spasm of the cardiac sphincter – cardiospasm or *achalasia* (Gr. chaleo = to loosen). This occurs mostly in middle-aged women, in whom the nerve cells of the oesophageal plexus atrophy so that there is gradual failure of relaxation of the sphincter and corresponding hesitation in the food entering the stomach. Both of the above are uncommon causes of dysphagia, more frequently it is caused by a hiatus hernia, a foreign body of some kind or a carcinoma.

Hiatus hernia and the accompanying reflux of acid (*reflux oesophagitis*) is probably the commonest cause of oesophageal problems, and consists of herniation of the upper part of the stomach through a hiatus or gap in the diaphragm which may be unnaturally weak or subject to exceptional pressure from obesity, pregnancy etc. This may be symptomless in some people but in others leads to disruption of the cardiac sphincter with corresponding reflux of acid from the stomach which may regurgitate into the mouth and even spill over into the lungs and lead to persistant episodes of chest infection. Since the oeso-phagus is not designed to withstand acidity there is a painful sensation (heartburn) and sometimes ulceration of the mucous membrane of the lower oesophagus.

The reflux is worst when the patient stoops, lifts or lies down, especially after a big meal. Conversely loosening tight clothing, propping the head of the bed on bricks and taking alkaline fluids relieve the symptoms. Hiccoughs may sometimes be a problem due to stimulation of the diaghragm, and occasionally the hernia is so large that it actually compresses the lung and causes dyspnoea. Complications from a hiatus hernia arise from the ulceration of the oesophagus which oozes blood and may lead to anaemia if iron stores are deficient. Or it may heal with much scarring and fibrosis with a resulting stricture and dysphagia.

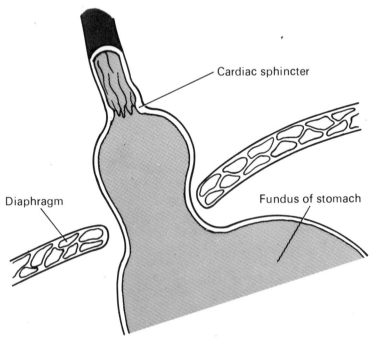

Cardiac sphincter

Diaphragm

Fundus of stomach

Fig. 12.1   *Hiatus hernia*

Oesophageal cancer occurs mostly in elderly men, especially smokers, and has a poor prognosis as it rapidly ulcerates through the wall and spreads to other structures. The lower part of the oesophagus is where it tends to occur and where the dysphagia is noted, first for solids and then later for liquids also. It is extremely common in some parts of the world especially China, owing to the high temperature at which food is swallowed and the high content of spices and moulds found in the diet.

The Stomach

The necessity of the stomach to secrete acid is also its main weakness when the resistance of the mucosa fails. The result is *peptic ulceration* and this may occur in the *stomach, oesophagus* or *duodenum*. The exact cause has long been a source of speculation, but factors such as dental decay, diet, smoking, alcohol and particularly emotional stress all play a part. Recently there has been evidence that infection by bacteria of the Campylobacter species occurs in a large proportion of cases.

Gastric ulcers are ulcers of the lining of the stomach often located on the lesser curvature near the pylorus (see figure 12.2). They are found particularly in men and women from economically and socially deprived areas, especially in Scotland and the North of England, and tend to be chronic and recur every few weeks as a flare-up in the continuous background of gnawing epigastric pain, especially after an alcoholic drink. The pain is also characteristically worse after eating, when acid is secreted, so the sufferers are usually thin and avoid food or vomit it up which brings relief. Mutiple tiny ulcers called *gastric erosions* are seen sometimes as side-effects of some drugs, particularly aspirin, cortisone and the anti-inflammatory drugs which all may cause bleeding.

Duodenal ulcers on the other hand are seen mostly in younger men in high-pressured, stressful careers ('executive ulcers'), and in many cases there is an excessive secretion of acid by the stomach. Women are largely immune from these ulcers, possibly for hormonal reasons. The pain is identical in quality to that of a gastric ulcer but tends to be present several hours after a meal when the stomach is empty, sometimes waking the patient in the small hours of the morning as a 'hunger-pain'. Relief is usually sought by eating bland food or drinking milk, so they may put on weight and look surprisingly well-nourished.

Peptic ulcers may come and go quite quickly, resembling aphthous ulcers in this respect, but some run a prolonged course for months and even years. Some even develop complications, the main ones being as follows:

—*Bleeding*. This may be very heavy if an artery is eroded, and the stomach or duodenum fills with blood which may be vomited (*haematemesis*). If the blood has been in the stomach for a while, the acid will oxidise it to a dark brown material with the appearance of coffee grounds. In some the blood first appears in the stools as tarry black *melaena* (Gr. melanos = black) which has a characteristic, rather pungent odour. Both haematemesis and melaena signify bleeding fairly high in the digestive tract, not necessarily from an ulcer. Other possibilities are from an *erosion*

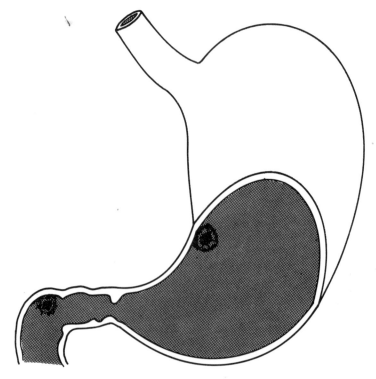

Fig. 12.2   *Typical sites for gastric and duodenal ulcer*

in the stomach, usually due to aspirin or similar drugs, from a *stomach tumour* or from leaking *oesophageal varices* (see chapter 14).

—*Perforation*. Few ulcers are severe enough to penetrate into the peritoneal cavity, but occasionally one does, especially if the patient is taking steroids, and the result is that acid flows out and causes a chemical *peritonitis*. The first evidence of this is a sudden, excruciating pain in the upper abdomen which is aggravated by the slightest movement. Because the diaphragm is often involved the pain may be felt in the shoulders but will cause the patient to lie absolutely *motionless*. Even the bowels cease their peristalsis and the result is complete silence of the bowel sounds, later with distension as air finds its way into the peritoneum. After a few hours the patient is liable to become shocked and require an operation, when the perforation is plugged with a convenient piece of omentum.

—*Stenosis*. Narrowing of the pylorus or even the lower part of the stomach may occur in the case of an ulcer which has healed repeatedly with much scarring and fibrosis. If peristalsis is unable to urge food through, the stomach will dilate until it is two or three times its normal size, and then vomit up old food eaten one or two days before. Obviously the patient will lose weight rapidly and become thin and undernourished, so this situation is often mistaken for cancer.

Congenital pyloric stenosis, though unrelated to ulcers, is a similar situation occurring in some newborn babies who have a congenital hypertrophy of the pyloric muscle. The baby, usually a first-born male, begins to vomit its feeds at the age of 3–4 weeks and to lose weight. The vomitus emerge with great force ('projectile vomiting') a short while after the feed is over, and the baby is then immediately hungry again and demands another feed, only for the process to be repeated. Sometimes peristalsis may be visible through the abdominal wall, and the enlarged sphincter felt on palpation. If the situation does not settle an operation to widen the pylorus may be required.

Stomach Cancer

Gastric carcinoma has actually declined in Britain over the last 30 years but is still the third most common form of cancer in both men and women after lung, breast and colon. In some countries, e.g. Japan and Portugal, the incidence is 2–3 times as high as in

Britain and the US which suggests that dietary factors are involved, and the chief culprit is thought probably to be nitrate derivatives, some of which are highly carcinogenic. These take the form of nitrosamines which are derived through the combination of nitrites with amines in the food by gut organisms, and this reaction is blocked by vitamin C which thus has a protective effect.

Individuals with little or no acid in their stomachs (achlorhydria), a situation prevalent in pernicious anaemia and after gastrectomy, are at a much greater risk as the bacteria which perform the nitrosamine reaction are able to survive in the stomach. There is also a possibility that cimetidine, a drug much used to lower the acid content in the stomachs of ulcer patients, will have a similar effect. Moreover, we now have a situation where the quantities of nitrates used by modern farming as fertilizer are so great that the water table is becoming contaminated. Strangely, the incidence of cancer in the small intestine is extremely low, and no theory has adequately explained this. It may be that the very high turnover of cells which are continually being shed prevents abnormal tissue remaining long in the body, or perhaps that the secretions of the small bowel being so prolific the potential carcinogens are diluted.

Most cases of stomach cancer arise in the region of the pylorus, and hence obstruct the outflow and lead to nausea and discomfort after food. This symptom occurring in a 50–60 year old should arouse suspicion, and enquiry will often reveal *anorexia, weight loss* and vague *dyspepsia* or malaise. Eventually there will be vomiting of food similar to the pyloric stenosis following a gastric ulcer, and indeed a gastric ulcer, though not a duodenal, may sometimes become malignant. If the tumour is up at the cardiac end of the stomach, then the predominant symptom is likely to be dysphagia, and perhaps the appearance of a node in the supraclavicular area. A common accompanying feature is bleeding, which may pass unnoticed for a while until the patient becomes obviously pale and anaemic, by which time he may have metastatic spread to the lymph nodes and the liver, when jaundice is likely to ensue. So the terminal picture is that of extreme weight loss (*cachexia*), pallor, jaundice and ascites with a swollen peritoneum containing malignant cells. The prognosis is unfortunatly poor and only about 5% survive more than 5 years.

The Pancreas

This gland has two functions, the secretion of the hormones insulin and glucagon for the control of glucose metabolism, and the secretion of enzymes into the duodenum for digestion of fat, protein and carbohydrate. Failure of its first function of course produces diabetes, but fortunately this seldom affects enzyme production and digestion is not impaired. Less commonly the whole gland is affected by blockage, tumour or inflammation and the result is the passage of undigested fat in the stools – *steatorrhoea* (Gr. steatos = fat) and the inability to absorb nutrients from the small intestine – *malabsorption.*

Cystic fibrosis is the usual cause of blockage of the pancreatic ducts, and is due to an inherited defect in the glands of the body producing mucus, which is much too viscid and blocks the ducts, thus preventing the enzymes from emerging. A similar problem occurs in the lungs in this condition, and there is often chestiness and wheezing. The problem usually manifests soon after birth with constipation or steatorrhoea and a failure to thrive and develop normally. Depending on the thickness of the mucus, the child will be more or less affected but is likely to die prematurely and require supplements of pancreatic enzymes with each meal. Another feature is that the sweat is extremely salty, and this is used as the basis of a test used to confirm the diagnosis.

Cancer of the pancreas is a less common tumour of the gut but notoriously difficult to diagnose as it may present in a variety of different ways. This may be as *jaundice*, from blockage of the common bile duct, as vague dyspeptic symptoms such as nausea, vomiting and anorexia, or as a dull pain in the upper abdomen often radiating through to the back, relieved by bending double. Sometimes there is an inexplicable fever, or phlebitis which moves around the body ('thrombophlebitis migrans'). There is a possible link between the incidence of pancreatic carcinoma and a high consumption of coffee.

Pancreatitis is an inflammation of the pancreas and may be either acute or chronic in its onset. The acute type is caused by the pancreas suddenly digesting itself with its own proteolytic enzymes (Gr. pan = all; kreas = meat). The reason for this is not known, but there is usually a history of either *gallstones* or *alcoholism*, and in most cases reflux of bile up the pancreatic duct.

The pain is severe and located in the epigastrium, coming on quickly and radiating through to the back, but typically eased by leaning forward. The patient looks and is very ill and shocked, and may develop jaundice. The chronic type of pancreatitis consists of fibrosis of the gland following repeated acute attacks or simply damage by alcohol. The pain is less severe but recurrent, especially after alcohol, and the patient will begin to lose weight and may even become diabetic if the Islets of Langerhans are involved.

13

Intestines: Disorders of Absorption

Small Intestine

Because almost all the nutrients are absorbed through the wall of the small intestine the most significant consequence of disorders of this organ is malabsorption, a feature common to allergic, infective and inflammatory conditions and leading to the passage of undigested food or steatorrhoea. If peristalsis is also affected there will be accompanying colicky pains and diarrhoea, sometimes with bleeding.

Coeliac disease is the main allergic cause of malabsorption and was first described in 1888 by Dr Gee of Gee's Linctus fame. His description was of infants who, soon after weaning, began to lose weight and pass frequent pale, bulky and offensive stools which floated on water. They were very miserable children with distended abdomens and emaciated limbs, later developing anaemia, bruising and dermatitis due to vitamin and iron deficiency. The condition occurred in about one child in 2000 and was generally fatal, but mysteriously disappeared during World War II in some countries, only to reappear afterwards. At length it was realized that a protein called *gluten* in wheat and other cereals was responsible, and that by excluding this from the diet the child recovered. Apparently these children were allergic to the gluten and suffered damage to the villi which atrophied and thereby the absorptive power of the gut was lost. A similar condition is found in adults who develop the emaciation and anaemia but not necessarily the steatorrhoea, indeed they often become constipated at the onset of the condition which is known as *adult coeliac disease*.

Crohn's disease is a somewhat more mysterious condition whose aetiology is unknown, though some suspect an allergic

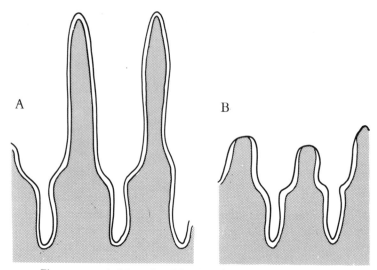

Fig. 13.1   *A. Normal and B. Atrophic villi of coeliac disease*

basis here too. Regions of the ileum, especially the terminal portion, become inflamed and oedematous, leaving normal bowel in between ('skip lesions'), which gives it the alternative name of *regional ileitis*. The areas affected by oedema develop deep cracks which give them a cobblestone appearance, and these fissures may extend through the wall of the bowel to join with other surfaces and form *fistulae*. This extension of the inflammation leads to tangled, adherent loops of bowel known as *adhesions*, and it is these that are responsible for a lot of the colicky pain which the disease causes.

The condition starts quite suddenly in teenagers or young adults, with pain in the lower abdomen, fever and diarrhoea, so it is easily mistaken for appendicitis. There is usually an inflamed mass of tender bowel palpable in the right iliac fossa, and this may even cause an obstruction to the bowel and severe colic. The disease may resolve itself in a few weeks or run a chronic course with recurrent episodes for months or years and lead to complications. These include *malabsorption* and *anaemia, fistula formation, strictures* and *obstruction*. Because the whole body is involved symptoms outside the bowel such as clubbing of the fingers, arthritis, uveitis and ankylosing spondylitis are not uncommon.

Infections by bacteria, viruses and protozoa as well as infestations by parasites may lead to malabsorption under certain circumstances, especially if they become chronic. These are described in chapter 3 in the section on gastroenteritis.

Appendix

This has long been thought of as a vestigial organ with only a nuisance value when it malfunctions. However it does contain a large amount of lymphoid tissue and may play an important part in fighting infection, a sort of 'tonsil of the intestine'. Like the tonsils it is most active between the ages of 2 and 20, and this is the age when appendicitis is most likely to occur. And like the tonsil it may inflame and even form an appendix abscess, the equivalent of a quinsy, but since it is not visible, the safest procedure has always been appendicectomy.

The first symptom of appendicitis is pain, generally colicky and in the umbilical region. The person feels nauseous and may vomit, and may sometimes get dysuria if the appendix happens to lie over the ureter, which is rather misleading. There is usually a slight fever and furred tongue with foul breath at this point, and the pain then usually localises halfway between the umbilicus and the iliac crest on the right – *McBurney's point* – which indicates that the appendix is acutely inflamed and likely to perforate. There will be tenseness of the abdominal muscles, and pain if they are pressed gently and then released, *rebound tenderness*.

Appendicitis either resolves, and this may happen many times in a so-called 'grumbling appendix', or goes on to perforate, in which case an *appendix abscess* will usually form. This is allowed to settle down for several weeks and then either drained or removed. Occasionally a ruptured appendix is followed by the spread of pus throughout the peritoneal cavity and generalised *peritonitis* results.

Large Intestine

Here water is absorbed from the stools, at a rate which depends on the speed of flow of the products of digestion through the colon. Thus excessive peristaltic activity will lead to diarrhoea, and delay to constipation. The former is symptomatic of most inflammatory conditions and if these are very severe may be accompanied by the passage of fresh blood. Diarrhoea may also be caused by anxiety, malabsorption and thyrotoxicosis, as well as by local pathology.

Constipation, the infrequent passage of hard stools, is likely to occur particularly in those who consume a so-called 'low residue' diet which contains little roughage or fibre. This gives little stimulus to the bowel which becomes sluggish, and is especially a problem in the elderly whose muscles are weak. In them, and in some children who are reluctant to move their bowels, large quantities of faeces build up and impact so that finally they become incontinent. Constipation also occurs during a pyrexial illness, dehydration from any cause, obstruction by a carcinoma or any other cause, hypothyroidism and in those who avoid defaecation on account of pain from piles or an anal fissure.

Colitis

Colitis is to the large intestine what enteritis is to the small, that is to say it refers generally to inflammatory conditions characterised by pain and diarrhoea (sometimes an infection of both is referred to as an 'enterocolitis'). There are two types of colitis, ulcerative colitis and what used to be called mucous colitis but is now more commonly known as irritable bowel or spastic colon.

Irritable bowel syndrome is a common disorder of the lower bowel whereby the regular waves of peristalsis become unco-ordinated and generate colicky pains, diarrhoea and constipation. The stools often contain an excessive amount of mucus and sometimes there is much flatulence with abdominal distension and fearful rumblings ('borborygmi'). Not uncommonly the need to hurry to the toilet arises after meals, especially breakfast, and the person is then well for the rest of the day. The pains are dull and cramplike, and may be felt anywhere in the abdomen which can be confusing, but most often in the left iliac fossa. The condition is more common in women than in men, especially those of an anxious disposition, and is seen between the ages of 20–40. What is conspicuously absent is the evidence of serious consequences such as anaemia, weight loss or bleeding, and the general health is usually good.

The causes of irritable bowel are uncertain, but emotional factors play a part, and this is in many ways the female equivalent of a duodenal ulcer with its occurrence in tense, overconscientious people, often with exacerbations before a period. Food sensitivity also plays a large part and it may be of benefit to exclude such substances as wheat, milk and other dairy foods, tea, coffee and oranges from the diet. It is also possible that Candida infection may play some part by damaging the bowel wall and permitting allergens to enter in large quantities.

Ulcerative colitis is altogether a more serious form of colitis involving especially the descending colon and rectum (the latter is termed a *proctitis*). It is relatively common among younger adults in their 20s and 30s, but the cause is unknown. One theory is that it is a result of an abnormal response by the immune system to a strain of E. coli organisms which reside in the lower bowel, for many of the patients possess autoantibodies against their own bowel mucosa. In some cases there is considerable improvement from avoiding milk and dairy products, and this should be tried. Whatever the cause, the result is a series of extensive ragged ulcers in the wall of the colon which leave areas of normal, swollen tissue between which are known as 'pseudopolyps'.

As might be expected the main symptoms are abdominal pain and diarrhoea accompanied by bleeding and thin mucus which oozes from the ulcers, and this leads rapidly to dehydration and anaemia in a severe case. The diarrhoea characteristically continues through the night, which helps to identify its cause, and it is accompanied by a fever and rapid loss of weight during an acute attack. Most of these episodes pass within a few days or weeks, but may relapse at any time. Occasionally an ulcer becomes deep enough to perforate the wall and cause peritonitis which is extremely serious, or the bowel becomes paralysed and bowel sounds cease ('toxic dilatation'). In this case it may be necessary to operate and create a *colostomy*, which involves making an artificial anus by bringing the bowel out on to the abdominal wall and allowing the unused part to recover. In some the disease persists as ill health and constant diarrhoea from a bowel that has partly healed but become scarred and rigid, sometimes leading to strictures. Another complication which may occur after a number of years is malignant change in the bowel wall and bowel cancer is more common in those with ulcerative colitis. Like Crohn's disease a number of systemic complications may arise in the course of time, the main ones being arthritis and skin problems.

Diverticular Disease

Western society has over the past century progressively refined its diet so that much of the fibre has been removed, and this leads to constipation as the bulk of the stools is reduced and the pressure required for peristalsis is correspondingly increased. A consequence of this is that the wall of the colon is liable to give way at its weakest point, this being at the side, where the blood vessels enter, and the result is the formation of small sacs or diverticuli. These are often present unknowingly in the elderly, a condition known as *diverticulosis*, and no great harm is done unless one of them becomes blocked and inflamed, which usually happens in the pelvic part of the colon and is then called *diverticulitis*.

Fig. 13.2   *Diverticuli in descending and sigmoid colon*

A condition very similar to that of appendicitis results, and indeed the symptoms are virtually identical but on the left side of the abdomen. Initially there is colicky pain and then later an abscess may form which will cause a fever and a tender mass in the left iliac fossa which may go on to rupture. Because the site of the abscess is at the entry of the blood vessel, heavy *rectal bleeding* may be the first sign of the disease, and there will often be either diarrhoea or constipation and sometimes even obstruction of the bowel. These symptoms are also extremely similar to those of a carcinoma of the colon, and as both conditions occur in the same age group the diagnosis is often difficult.

Bowel Cancer

Cancer of the colon is the commonest cancer of the digestive tract in Western countries, and there is considerable evidence that this relates not only to the relative lack of fibre in the diet but to the large amounts of protein and to a lesser extent fat which are acted upon by the bowel bacteria to create potential carcinogens. Possibly on account of this, two thirds of the cancers occur in the terminal part of the colon – the sigmoid and the rectum, which may be just as well since they are diagnosed more early here because they are more likely to lead to an obstruction and call attention to themselves. Conditions which predispose to malignant change include longstanding *ulcerative colitis* (at one time the bowel was removed prophylactically), the presence of *polyps* in the colon and the removal of the gallbladder.

The symptoms are either *rectal bleeding* (which is liable to be dismissed as piles), a change in bowel habit to either constipation or diarrhoea, or a dull ache in the left iliac fossa or lower abdomen. Cancer of the ascending colon seldom causes an obstruction until it has been present for some time, and as the early symptoms are vague the prognosis is correspondingly worse. Eventually spread occurs to the local lymphatics, to the liver causing enlargement and *jaundice*, and to the peritoneum causing *ascites*.

Rectum and Anus

Haemorrhoids, or *piles* as they are more commonly known, are

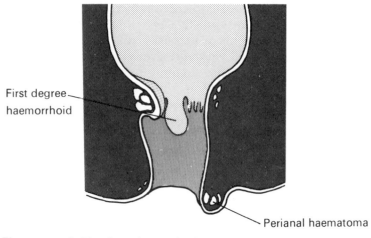

First degree
haemorrhoid

Perianal haematoma

Fig. 13.3   *A. First degree haemorrhoids in upper anal canal, with a perianal haematoma.*

varicose veins of the anal margin and as such have similar causes to those of the leg. Most cases occur spontaneously due to an inherited weakness but some follow compression such as that caused by pregnancy, constipation or even a tumour. The first symptom of piles is usually itching or bleeding. Blood is noticed when the bowels are moved (haemorrhoids means 'flowing blood'), sometimes in quite large quantities, and if this continues the patient may even develop iron deficiency anaemia. The attack of piles may clear up or progress to form swellings which prolapse outside the anal margin (*second degree piles*) during

Protruding pile

B. Third degree haemorrhoids.

defaecation but are usually replaced by the patient afterwards for comfort. If they remain outside the anal margin like the proverbial bunch of grapes then their blood supply is likely to be cut off and they are then said to be *strangulated piles* or 'third degree haemorrhoids', and an extremely painful condition that is! Eventually they turn a dark shade of purple and atrophy after 2–3 weeks and vanish, leaving only a small tag of skin as a reminder.

Other anal conditions are sometimes mistaken for an attack of piles, and these are:

—*Anal fissure:* a small crack, usually at the posterior margin of the anus which may appear after the passage of a hard stool, and persist for some time to cause pain and constipation.

— *Peri-anal haematoma*: a small cherry-red lump appears suddenly at the anal margin after straining, looking very like a pile but due to sudden rupture of a vein. It is painful but subsides within a few days.

— *Anal fistula*: a fistula is an abnormal communication between two mucosal surfaces, and at the anus this may occur from Crohn's disease or sometimes after an abscess at the anal margin.

— *Rectal dyschezia*: a mysterious condition characterised by sudden, severe, neuralgic pain of the rectum, anus or even genitalia and occurring spontaneously or occasionally during orgasm. It subsides after a few seconds with no ill-effects but is extremely distressing. The cause is unknown. (Gr. kezo = to ease oneself, i.e. to move one's bowels).

14

Liver: Disorders of Manufacture and Destruction

The function of the liver, the largest gland in the body, can be likened to that of an enormous factory where raw materials enter and are converted, stored and finally despatched or broken down with the aid of innumerable enzymes. Infection or destruction of the liver will thus affect a very large number of different functions, as will blockage of the inflow or outflow tracts, and diseases of the liver reflect this by causing enlargement (*hepatomegaly*), destruction of the cells (*cirrhosis*), overflow of bile into the blood (*jaundice*) or obstruction to the flow of blood in the portal system (*portal hypertension*), either singly or combined.

Hepatomegaly

The liver is not normally palpable, being well hidden up under the ribs, and if it can be felt this indicates that all is not well (except in the case of young babies whose liver is working overtime to synthesize protein for growth and break down foetal blood cells, and is therefore normally palpable). The usual reasons for enlargement are *hepatitis, cirrhosis* or *tumour*, and occasionally certain blood disorders or chronic infections.

Acute viral hepatitis is the commonest liver disease and is an enormous problem worldwide, being related very largely to standards of hygiene and sanitation. Viral infections of the liver can occur with glandular fever and yellow fever, but the term 'viral hepatitis' is used to refer to that caused by a group of three viruses known as hepatitis A, B and 'non A, non B' (see below). In all three types the symptoms are very similar though there are differences in the outcome and mode of transmission.

Hepatitis A, which also goes by the name of *infectious hepatitis*, has an incubation period of about 2-6 weeks and is spread by the oral-faecal route especially among the young, so small epidemics appear in schools and institutions from time to time. The symptoms come on over a few days as a fever with marked *anorexia, nausea, diarrhoea* and upper *abdominal discomfort,* the liver being enlarged and tender. Soon a faint tinge of *jaundice* will usually, but not always, appear and the stools go pale, but this seldom lasts more than a week or two although the itching of the skin which sometimes accompanies it may linger and full recovery take many months. Damage to the liver is rarely severe but alcohol should be avoided for a year.

Hepatitis B or *serum hepatitis* is spread by direct contact with the blood, saliva or semen of an infected person or a carrier, hence its occurrence in IV drug addicts, homosexual or bisexual men (for reasons similar to AIDs), and those working in dialysis units. It is also considerably more likely to occur in immigrants from Africa, Asia or the Mediterranean. The incubation period is longer, 2–6 months, and the disease is seen mostly in young men as opposed to schoolchildren. The onset is slower but the symptoms more severe than type A, often with arthritis and a considerable degree of jaundice, and the infection may persist for a long time, some patients even remaining carriers of the virus when they have recovered. In order to confirm the diagnosis the blood is examined for evidence of the viral antigen, known as 'Australia antigen' because it was first discovered in the blood of an aborigine. The immediate outlook for hepatitis B is good, but in the long term there is a high incidence of cirrhosis or liver cancer.

Hepatitis non A non B, a somewhat clumsy title which merely indicates that as yet the agent(s) are unknown, is a waterborne disease found especially in India with a degree of severity somewhere between the other two.

Cirrhosis

The word comes from the Greek meaning 'tawny', and refers to the greyish-brown discoloration which the liver undergoes when its cells are injured and the original architecture of the delicate lobules is replaced by a scarred battleground of fibrous tissue. Cirrhosis is classically associated with longstanding *alcoholism,* but may also appear after *hepatitis* or as a result of *heart failure.* A particular type of cirrhosis, occurring mostly in women, arises as a result of sluggishness in the flow of bile due to an autoimmune connective tissue disorder – *primary biliary cirrhosis*.

Most of these causes start by inflaming the liver and making it swell in a variety of different ways, and each has a specific pathological characteristic when seen under a microscope. So the liver may start as a swollen, 'fatty liver' but then gradually shrinks as fibrosis overtakes the attempts at regeneration and finally ends up as a shrivelled 'nodular liver'. Naturally, many functions of the liver are affected and in the extreme case may fail altogether – *liver failure* or 'hepatocellular failure' – and this is the endpoint of several different kinds of liver disorders. There are simply not enough cells left to carry out the functions of the organ, and a number of clinical features ensue:

—wasting, due to the inability to form proteins.
—ascites (Gr. askos = a wineskin) due to the low plasma proteins (the presence of proteins in the plasma normally draws fluid out of the tissues by osmosis).
—spider naevi, due to dilation of the capillaries in the skin of the face and neck.
—gynaecomastia (male breast enlargement), due to inability to break down sex hormones, particularly oestrogens.
—testicular atrophy and impotence for the same reasons.
—jaundice, due to failure of bilirubin metabolism.
—portal hypertension (see below).
—eventually coma and death from the build up of toxic waste especially ammonia.

Portal Hypertension

You will recall that the liver has blood delivered to it by both the hepatic artery, supplying oxygen, and the portal vein, supplying the products of digestion directly from the digestive tract lying within the peritoneum. If the branches of the portal vein become blocked, as may happen either through a tumour or cirrhosis, the back-pressure will start to cause oedema and engorgement of the gut, much in the way that left ventricular failure engorges the lungs. This means that the abdominal organs will swell up considerably, especially the spleen to cause enlargement of that organ (*splenomegaly*) and the blood will be forced into alternative routes.

There are three of these alternatives – the oesophageal vein at the top of the system, the haemorrhoidal vein at the bottom and the long defunct umbilical vein at the centre. All these have potential connections with the rest of the venous circulation and can be used to re-route the blood back to the heart. This means that the patient with portal hypertension will start to develop *piles* and swollen *oesophageal varices,* distended varicose veins in the lower oesophagus near the cardiac sphincter, the rupture of which is followed by a torrential haemorrhage and haema-temesis. If the umbilical vein is called into use then a delta of distended veins may be seen radiating from the umbilicus – the so-called Medusa's head or 'caput Medusae'.

Jaundice

In this state the small amount of bile which we normally have circulating in our blood is increased to the point where it becomes visible first in the sclera and then in the skin. This increase may be due to one of three reasons (see figure 14.1):

—the red cells are being broken down in numbers too great for the liver to cope. This is *haemolytic* or *pre-hepatic jaundice.*
—the liver cells are damaged and cannot conjugate the bile salts, *hepatocellular jaundice.*
—there is a blockage in the bile duct preventing outflow, *obstructive* or *post-hepatic jaundice.*

Haemolytic jaundice is uncommon except in certain blood disorders such as sickle-cell anaemia, thalassaemia, pernicious anaemia and rhesus disease, or in malaria. The jaundice is seldom very severe as the liver can cope with most of the bilirubin, but the simultaneous presence of anaemia gives these patients a characteristic lemon-yellow tinge.

Hepatocellular jaundice has already been mentioned in association with viral hepatitis, and there are many other agents which will damage the liver cells, particularly alcohol and drugs such as paracetamol, largactil and some antidepressants, as well as poisons such as phosphorus and the amanita fungi. These often have the effect of swelling the tissues which obstructs the outflow of what bile is formed, a situation called 'biliary stasis'. A similar situation arises in the familiar *neonatal jaundice,* when the immature liver is unable to conjugate the large amount of bilirubin because its enzymes have not yet fully formed. This is therefore sometimes aided by stimulating similar enzymes in the skin by using UV light in order to prevent a build-up of bilirubin which might deposit in the brain and cause a form of

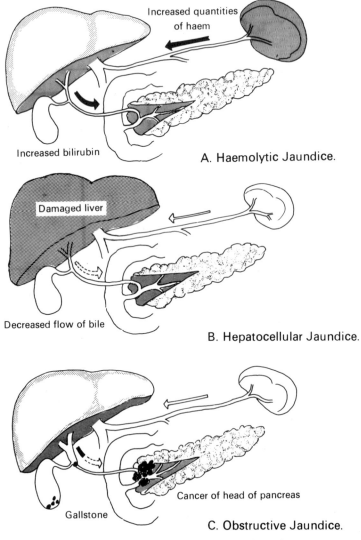

Increased quantities of haem

Increased bilirubin

A. Haemolytic Jaundice.

Damaged liver

Decreased flow of bile

B. Hepatocellular Jaundice.

Cancer of head of pancreas

Gallstone

C. Obstructive Jaundice.

Fig. 14.1   *The different causes of jaundice*

damage termed *kernicterus* ('icterus' means jaundiced and Kera was the goddess of destruction).

Obstructive jaundice arises as a result either of compression of the bile duct by a tumour, or from a gallstone. As no bile flows there is an increasingly deepening level of jaundice with pale clay-coloured stools and dark urine. The circulating bile leads to itching of the skin and a metallic taste in the mouth, and if a stone is present there will usually be colicky pain.

Tumours arising in the liver are known as *hepatomas*, and are rare in this country but the commonest cancer on a worldwide basis. Most Western cancers obstructing bile outflow are found to arise in the head of the pancreas, or more commonly as secondary tumours coming from the colon or stomach which swell the lymphatics at the exit of the bile duct from the liver.

Gallstones are discussed in detail in the next section.

Gallstones

This common condition increases in frequency with age, but does so more rapidly in women so that young women are more likely to suffer from *cholelithiasis*, as stones are sometimes called, than young men but the incidence evens up later on. Oestrogens appear to be a factor as gallstones are associated with having children, diabetes and taking the contraceptive pill, and there is still a modicum of truth in the adage about the 'fair, fat, fertile and flatulent'. A highly refined carbohydrate diet is another factor, as the synthesis of cholesterol in the bile is increased, but the question of what exactly causes gallstones has no simple answer, and there is more than a single cause as although the majority of stones contain cholesterol a few consist only of bile pigments.

Because the chief function of the gallbladder is to concentrate bile by a factor of about twelve times there is always a risk that cholesterol, the main bile salt, will crystallise and form a nucleus around which other substances can deposit. The majority of those with stones in the gallbladder do not know it as they have no symptoms. Some get a vague feeling of discomfort and flatulence, particularly after a fatty meal, called 'flatulent dyspepsia', but this may happen for other reasons also, such as hiatus hernia. An unfortunate minority suffer from more severe consequences such as biliary colic or cholecystitis.

Biliary colic is the name given to the pain which accompanies the passage of a stone down the bile duct. This may happen when the gallbladder contracts after a meal, causing a sudden pain in the epigastrium which becomes steadily worse with sweating, vomiting and extreme restlessness. It is felt mainly in the upper abdomen but may also radiate to the lower end of the right scapula or the shoulder tip, and continues steadily for some hours, ceasing only when the stone has passed into the duodenum. If the stone takes more than a few hours to pass then the resulting obstruction to bile leads to a degree of jaundice with pale stools and darkening of the urine.

In some the stone becomes impacted in the neck of the gallbladder and leads to pain after meals when the gland contracts, and also to stagnation of the bile which cannot escape. This state of affairs will eventually end with the bile becoming infected and causing an acute inflammation or *cholecystitis*, with fever, malaise and tenderness over the liver, sometimes with a tinge of jaundice if the duct is also inflamed. This may be a recurrent situation every time the patient consumes fatty food, and eventually the gallbladder will become shrivelled, function-less and liable to malignancy, and is therefore often removed by the operation of 'cholecystectomy'.

15

Kidney: Disorders of Excretion

The predominant function of the kidney is to maintain a constant internal water and mineral balance, and to eliminate waste and surplus material. Its huge powers of filtration and secretion allow the kidney to monitor the volume, acidity, toxicity and mineral content of the whole circulation every 30 minutes or so, for one fifth of the output from the heart travels down the renal arteries. This means that the function of the renal tubules is vital, and although we possess a large reserve and can even manage on a single kidney, diseases of the substance or *parenchyma* of the kidney may damage the delicate filtration in one of three main ways. These are, very broadly speaking, through inflammation of the filter (*nephritis*), by perforation of the filter with 'holes' (*nephrosis*), and by total blockage of the filter (*renal failure*).

As well as this constant adjustment of the blood, two other important functions related to this are performed by the kidney. These are the control of blood pressure by the hormone renin which the glomerular cells secrete, and the stimulation of erythrocyte production by the secretion of erythropoietin in response to anoxia, and both these mechanisms may go awry and lead to hypertension, anaemia or even polycythaemia.

A variety of terms are used in describing renal disease, the main ones being as follows:

—*Anuria*: absence of urinary output from the kidney.
—*Retention*: inability to pass urine present in the bladder.
—*Oliguria*: passage of scanty urine from the kidney.
—*Polyuria*: passage of large quantities of urine ('diuresis').
—*Haematuria*: passing blood in the urine.
—*Glycosuria*: passing glucose in the urine.
—*Proteinuria*: passing protein in the urine (=albuminuria).
—*Dysuria*: painful passage of urine.

—*Incontinence*: involuntary passage of urine.
—*Micturition*: the act of urination.
—*Strangury*: constant urge to urinate but with the painful passage of only one or two drops of (bloodstained) urine.

Acute Glomerulonephritis (Nephritis)

In 1827 Richard Bright gave a classic description of a disease he called 'acute nephritis', and which has since come to be known as Bright's disease or acute glomerulonephritis (AGN). He noticed that some children develop a feverish illness with a puffy face and pain in the loins about 2 weeks after a sore throat or attack of tonsillitis. The urine is scanty (oliguria) and either bloodstained or discoloured and smoky, depending on the amount of haematuria, and the blood pressure is moderately elevated. Most of these children recover fully within a week or so, and this recovery is announced by a diuresis with a marked polyuria, but a few have a prolonged period of anuria, sometimes lasting 4–6 weeks.

From subsequent investigations it seems that certain strains of streptococci and occasionally other organisms provoke an antibody reaction by the immune system, and that these antibodies go on to damage the cells lining Bowman's capsule, which have a similar antigenic structure, resulting in their inflammation. Since Bright's time the advent of the electron microscope has enabled the distinction of many different types of changes in the glomeruli to be made, and this has lead to a complex classification of nephritis, such as 'proliferative', 'membranous' etc, but all have the features of *haematuria, proteinuria, oedema* and *oliguria*.

One particular variety of glomerulonephritis which is due to an allergic reaction to an unknown agent is 'Henoch-Schonlein purpura'. It is seen in children after an acute fever, and they develop a purpuric (haemorrhagic) rash on the legs and buttocks, with pains and swellings in the joints, abdominal colic and even bleeding from the bowel in addition to the nephritis.

Renal Failure

When the kidneys fail they are no longer able to secrete urine, and hence the main constituents – water, salt and urea – build up in the blood causing *oedema, hypertension* and *uraemia*. Urea is extremely toxic to the body and by the end of a week the patient was usually in a coma before the advent of dialysis and kidney machines, and died within a fortnight (much more rapidly than was the case with nephritis where the kidneys held out for weeks even in a severe case).

Renal failure may occur very suddenly if the blood supply is abruptly shut off as may happen after a heart attack, haemo-rrhage or severe dehydration. This is known as *acute renal failure*, and happens because the kidney tubules die in large numbers ('tubular necrosis'). A similar result happens when the tubules are poisoned by certain drugs, particularly some antibiotics like streptomycin, or after severe burns or crush injuries where large amounts of tissue are destroyed. There is then complete *anuria* and in order to slow down the rate of accumulation of urea it is important that the patient restricts the amount of protein consumed to a bare minimum, and also the amount of fluid drunk so they do not become 'waterlogged'. The symptoms of anorexia, nausea, vomiting, headache and hiccough increase unless the level of urea in the blood is lowered either spontaneously or by dialysis.

Damage to the kidney by diabetes mellitus, hypertension, infection (pyelonephritis), polycystic disease and sometimes renal stones, may lead to failure of the kidneys of a rather more leisurely sort, *chronic renal failure*. Here sufficient urine is passed but the concentrating power of the kidney is lost, so it is very dilute and tends to occur at night (*nocturia*). Because the production of erythropoietin is damaged there is almost always a degree of anaemia present too, and this condition runs a steady downhill course so it is these patients who are most likely to be offered renal transplants.

Nephrotic Syndrome (Nephrosis)

Some cases of nephritis never really recover and the glomeruli, despite patching themselves up after the inflammation, remain 'leaky'. This means that the larger molecules in the plasma will start to escape, especially the plasma proteins, the smaller globulins at first and then even the larger albumin. So the hallmark of nephrotic syndrome is *proteinuria*, and very large amounts of albumen and globulins may be lost to the body which make the urine cloudy so it froths up in the toilet. More seriously, the liver cannot synthesize albumen fast enough to keep pace with the loss, even though the patient is on a high protein diet, and so the plasma protein level begins to drop.

This has two major consequences; firstly the patient becomes very oedematous, often with *ascites*, because the plasma proteins are needed to maintain the osmotic pressure of the blood, and secondly they lack sufficient immunoglobulins to withstand infections which are therefore frequent. The typical clinical picture is a pale, anaemic individual who is swollen and oedematous but whose muscles are actually wasted because they lack protein, and who tends to suffer from repeated infectious illness. Not all cases of nephrotic syndrome are a result of glomerulonephritis, for sometimes diabetes mellitus and systemic lupus (SLE) may cause it, as may treatment with gold injections for rheumatoid arthritis.

Renal Stones and Obstruction

Stones or calculi are formed from crystals of substances present in urine which precipitate either because the urine is very concentrated, as occurs in chronic unaccustomed dehydration (the troops in North Africa during the last war frequently developed renal calculi) or because abnormal substances are present. These take the form of *calcium* salts which are excreted in large quantities when the patient is immobilised or drinks large amounts of milk, *uric acid* stones which may form in gout and *phosphate* stones in the presence of renal infection. It must be said, however, that in most cases of renal stones no abnormal constituents of the diet or urine can be found, though stones are known to be rare in vegetarians.

Most renal stones form in the pelvis or calyces of the kidney, and enlarge slowly to cause a dull pain in the loin which is worse when the patient is jarred. The stone may on occasions reach a very large size, occupying the whole of the renal pelvis and branching into the calyces – a *staghorn calculus*. More commonly the stone will pass down the ureter when it is the size of a grape seed, producing as it does the agony of *renal colic*. This is a sharp, severe pain which is referred from the loin down into the groin and testis (stones are much more common in men) and causing much restlessness in the patient as well as nausea, vomiting and sweating as he rolls about the bed. The pain is continuous and periodically increases in severity as the stone is squeezed a little further down the ureter, until it is eventually released into the bladder, from where there is little trouble passing it. The urine will be scanty and bloodstained, and sometimes infection will set in if the obstruction has been present for more than a few days.

At one time bladder stones were common in this country, and created chronic cystitis and severe strangury, as those familiar with the writings of Samuel Johnson will know. They appear to be a consequence of longstanding infection which may have been produced by the urethral strictures which follow untreated gonorrhoea, as well as to dietary factors which may explain the frequency of bladder stones in parts of Asia still.

Obstruction to the outflow of urine from the kidney not only leads to infection but may, if chronic, cause the pelvis and calyces to dilate and exert back-pressure on the tubules so that filtration can no longer occur. This situation is called a *hydronephrosis* and eventually the kidney becomes a cyst containing urine with little kidney substance left. The enlarged kidney may be palpable and there is often sediment in the urine and aching after drinking a lot of fluid, but the diagnosis is established by performing an intravenous pyelogram (IVP). This is the standard method of examining the kidney and ureters by injecting a radio-opaque dye into a vein which the kidney picks up and rapidly excretes, outlining the urinary tract on Xray as it does so and also giving a measure of its function. Stones will show up as small gaps in the dye as it flows down the ureter.

Polycystic disease is a similar condition affecting not only the kidneys but sometimes also the liver and pancreas as well. It is a congenital condition and when the kidneys are affected there are multiple cysts throughout its substance, some of which may be very large. The outcome depends on the amount of renal tissue which is damaged by pressure from the cysts, and whether renal failure, hypertension or infection supervene, any of which may shorten the life of the individual concerned.

Urinary Infections

Under normal circumstances the urinary tract is sterile, but some are susceptible to infections and these usually enter via the urethra from below and travel upwards, especially in the case of women as the urethra is short, straight and relatively wide. The invading organism is usually the commensal bacterium present in the gut, E. coli, which may sometimes exist in the bladder without causing symptoms, a situation called 'bacteriuria' and often occurring in pregnancy. More often, however, there is a sense of discomfort and frequency of micturition accompanied by dysuria and even strangury, the condition being called *cystitis* or *trigonitis*. The latter term is used if the symptoms are present without evidence of infection, as is the case in 50% of the women who suffer from recurrent dysuria, because the trigone of the bladder is constantly stimulated. This may result from trauma or allergy, and be worse after intercourse and if nylon tights or vaginal deodorants are used. Any condition causing stagnation of the flow of urine predisposes to infection, and it is thus commonly seen in pregnancy and where stones are present, when the infection is likely to ascend further and involve the kidney itself, causing pyelonephritis.

Acute pyelonephritis, sometimes called *pyelitis*, is an infection of the pelvis and deeper renal tissues and may occur without a previous cystitis, as happens quite often in pregnancy. The first symptoms are a sudden high *fever* with *rigors* (uncontrollable shivering), *aching in the loins* and usually nausea and *vomiting*. Both kidneys are generally involved and there is scanty, bloodstained urine containing pus cells. Some cases occur in children who develop recurrent attacks early in life either because they have a congenital abnormality in the valves of the bladder so the urine flows back up into the kidney as the bladder contracts during micturition, causing dilation and stagnation – *ureteric reflux.*

If the infection is not successfully eradicated then it may slowly penetrate into the parenchyma of the kidney and cause patchy areas of fibrosis and scarring of the nephrons so that over the years the kidney shrinks in size and *chronic pyelonephritis* results. There are recurrent bouts of loin pain and fever with slight dysuria, but eventually the renal function is compromised and hypertension develops.

Renal tuberculosis is an exception to the general rule of infection in that it starts in the kidney and spreads down the urinary tract to involve the bladder and epididymis especially. It is carried to the kidney in the blood from a primary focus in the lungs or gut, and causes the typical caseation which breaks through into a calyx and allows the organism to spread. There are no local symptoms, just the sweating and weight loss associated with TB, but examination of the urine reveals pus cells and red cells.

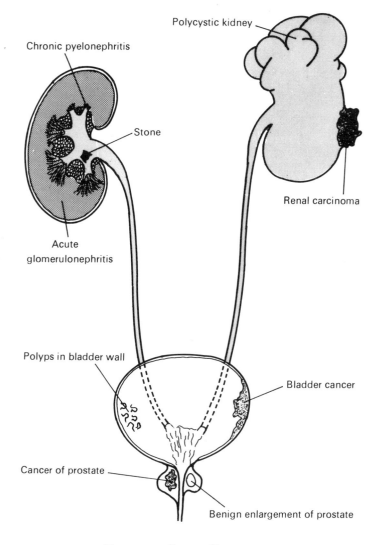

Fig. 15.1   *Causes of haematuria*

Tumours

The urinary tract is a place through which many chemicals, some of them potential carcinogens, are passed in high concentration, and it is therefore not surprising when either the kidney nephron or, more frequently, the lining of the bladder, undergoes neoplastic change.

Renal carcinomas arise in the delicate cells of the walls of the tubules and gradually compress the surrounding tissues before breaking out directly through the capsule of the kidney or spreading via the blood to a distant organ, often the lungs or bones. The earliest symptom is almost always *haematuria* which gives a grey tinge to the urine unless it is profuse, but sometimes a dragging pain in the loin develops or even a sudden renal colic from a clot of blood. Renal cancer is also notorious for causing a protracted malaise and intermittent fever for many weeks before it is discovered and should always be considered as a possibility in these circumstances.

The transitional cells which line the ureters and bladder are much more likely to develop malignant change than their renal counterparts, especially in those who smoke or consume large amounts of coffee. They arise as multiple warty growths called *papillomas* in middle-aged men, and in the early stages the epithelium is unstable but not as yet cancerous. However it is highly likely that one or more of these papillomas will eventually become invasive and infiltrate the wall of the bladder and surrounding tissues. Again, the first symptom is painless haematuria, sometimes with frequency. Later the tumour may obstruct the ureteric orifices and cause hydronephrosis of one of the kidneys. The conventional treatment of these papillomas is to remove them with a laser every few months as they occur.

16

Hormones: Disorders of Control

The function of the hormones is to maintain long term stabilization of the body's processes such as growth, metabolism and sex, the more immediate adjustments being left to the nervous system, although there are intimate connections between the two in the form of the 'hypothalamo-pituitary axis'. This means that disorders of the endocrine system are generally insidious in onset but have subtle and far-reaching affects. Although each pituitary hormone acts on a single tissue or organ, sometimes called a 'target organ', the hormones produced in turn by these target organs have a wide variety of activities which depend on a steady supply of the stimulating hormone, and most forms of pathology are therefore caused by an under or overproduction by these glands. The exception to this is diabetes mellitus, which is the commonest of all the hormonal disorders.

Pituitary Gland

This, the conductor of the whole glandular orchestra, is safely tucked away at the base of the brain, being accessible to the surgeon only via the upper recesses of the nose (L. pituita = a stuffy nose). It is responsible for the production of nine hormones, despite being only the size of a peanut, and damage to the gland therefore has very far-reaching consequences. Fortunately disorders are rare, although occasionally a benign tumour will cause oversecretion or infarction of the gland resulting in hypopituitarism.

Hypopituitarism, sometimes called 'Simmond's disease', is a loss of the secretions of the anterior pituitary usually as a result of a head injury or severe haemorrhage during labour, when the gland is most susceptible. The effect of this is the loss of hormones stimulating growth, sexual development, pigmentation and the thyroid and adrenal glands. In addition prolactin loss causes the milk to dry up in lactating mothers, and this may be the first sign. If the condition occurs before puberty the subject never grows up and remains, like Peter Pan, short and sexually underdeveloped.

Diabetes insipidus is another possible consequence of injury to the pituitary, but in this case it is the posterior lobe which is affected, resulting in a loss of antidiuretic hormone (ADH). This normally enables the kidney to conserve water by concentrating urine, so its absence results in the passage of large quantities of very dilute urine, up to four gallons a day. The main symptoms are thirst, nocturia and constipation, and the treatment usually involves taking synthetic ADH in the form of nasal drops.

Acromegaly is an example of overproduction of a pituitary hormone caused by a benign tumour (adenoma) in an adult. The hormone in question is growth hormone, and leads to enlargement of the hands, feet and jaw (Gr. acros = extremity) as well as the soft tissues. This results in a general coarsening of the features, a thick tongue, fatigue, aches and pains and increased sweating. Moreover the expanding tumour may give rise to headaches, and pressure on the nearby optic nerve lead to *defects in the visual field*. In the very rare event of the condition occurring in children it is known as giantism and the child or adolescent will start to develop exceptional stature if they are still in the growing phase. It is said that Goliath had just such a problem, and it was only his visual defect which enabled David to creep up on the blind side!

Thyroid Gland

Of all the glands under the influence of the pituitary, this is the one with the highest failure rate. When this happens the gland will often enlarge to form either a smooth (*diffuse*) or lumpy (*nodular*) swelling called a *goitre*. However, not all goitres are pathological and sometimes a so-called 'physiological goitre' is seen in normal pregnancy and in some adolescents. Goitres may result from a lack of iodine in the diet, or the consumption of excessive quantities of cabbage and similar vegetables which interfere with its uptake and are therefore termed 'goitrogens'. The thyroid is for some reason very susceptible to attack by antibodies, even those made erroneously by the body against itself (autoimmune disease), which may lead it to over or underproduce thyroxine and cause hyperthyroidism or hypothyroidism.

Hyperthyroidism or **thyrotoxicosis** occurs when the thyroid escapes control of the TSH from the pituitary and begins to produce increasing quantities of thyroxine under the influence of another hormone called 'long-acting thyroid stimulator' or LATS, which acts as a sort of 'counterfeit' TSH, while TSH itself is suppressed. LATS also causes enlargement of the pad of fat behind the eye, leading to the familiar bulging eyes or *exophthalmos* which is a noticeable feature of what is sometimes called *Grave's disease*.

It is most frequently seen in young women, who notice increasing exhaustion, nervousness, insomnia, sweating and palpitations, symptoms which might easily be put down to anxiety. The increasing amount of energy being metabolised is obtained by an enlarged appetite but with a paradoxical loss of weight, while tremor of the hands is caused by the bounding circulation which also leads to high blood pressure and even atrial fibrillation and dyspnoea. Peristalsis also increases and causes diarrhoea or more frequent normal stools, while the periods become scanty or cease altogether. The eyes feel inflamed and gritty, and double vision may occur if the muscles are affected.

Such a florid picture is seldom seen, and in older people the signs may be restricted to palpitations and wasting of the muscles, with no goitre or exophthalmos. In them it is often a small overactive *thyroid nodule* which is the problem, and this is another form of hyperthyroidism.

There are three conventional avenues of treatment – by antithyroid drugs, by removal of part of the gland (thyroidectomy) or by destruction of the gland with radioactive iodine. The drug treatment is normally tried first, but may result in relapse when the drug is stopped; surgery is the usual approach and works in the great majority but occasionally causes hypothyroidism which requires replacement with thyroxine, or a further relapse, when radioactive iodine may be recommended.

Hypothyroidism or **myxoedema** (Gr. myxos = mucus) can be a result of pituitary failure but is much more often due to damage to the thyroid itself by inflammation, drugs such as lithium, removal of too much of the gland for thyrotoxicosis or most often from an autoimmune process causing destruction of the gland, known as *Hashimoto's disease*. The term 'myxoedema' refers to the mucilaginous substance deposited under the skin giving it a puffy, yellow, coarse appearance, but differing from true oedema in that it does not pit under pressure. It is one of the commonest and most subtle of the endocrine disorders, arising usually in middle-aged women around the time of the menopause, and leading to weakness and fatigue, rheumatic pains and loss of appetite but not weight which may actually increase.

All bodily functions slow down, so there is apathy and poor memory, intellectual deterioration, slowing of the heart and possibly angina, sensitivity to the cold and increasing constipation. The hair thins and becomes lifeless, the voice deepens owing to deposits of myxoedema on the vocal chords, and there may be some deafness. Myxoedema compressing the median nerve in the wrist may lead to carpal tunnel syndrome with tingling of the fingers and a tendency to drop things. The periods become heavy and there is loss of interest in sex. Eventually, if not diagnosed and treated the condition terminates in coma preceded by paranoid delusions ('myxoedema madness').

Cretinism is the name sometimes given to hypothyroidism occurring in newborn babies whose thyroid gland fails to develop. Unless diagnosed and treated within a matter of weeks, the child will remain permanently dwarfed and mentally retarded (a cretin), so the condition should be suspected in all babies who are small, fail to feed well or are rather sluggish and underactive. Points to look for are the rather yellow complexion caused by carotene in the skin, a large, protruding tongue and umbilical hernia.

The Adrenal Glands

These glands are each actually double glands, one inside the other, each arising from different embryonic tissue. The central part, the medulla, derives from nervous tissue and secretes the hormones adrenalin and noradrenalin. It seldom malfunctions except in the very rare instance of a benign tumour secreting these substances in excess, called a 'phaeochromocytoma' (Gr. phaeos = gray; chromos = colour; cytos = cell). This causes paroxysms of sweating, palpitations, headache and hypertension along with a degree of panic from the rush of adrenalin. However, it is more commonly the cortex which malfunctions, either over or underproducing the hormone cortisone and leading to Cushing's syndrome or Addison's disease respectively (although both of these are rare).

Cushing's syndrome is a collection of symptoms arising from an excess of circulating steroid hormones in the body and is most commonly iatrogenic in origin when it is seen in those being treated with long-term cortisone for asthma, rheumatoid arthritis or one of the collagen diseases. It may also be caused by a tumour in the cortex stimulating overproduction of steroid hormones, or even in the pituitary causing excess ACTH secretion.

Whatever the cause, the symptoms are seen first in the face which becomes rounded and moon-shaped with reddening and acne. The trunk also swells and stretch marks and bruises appear on the skin. The fat over the shoulders increases and the bones become thin and brittle and the spine starts to collapse, leading to the familiar 'buffalo hump'. There is usually a rise in blood pressure, and because cortisone mobilises glucose from the cells of the liver, glycosuria appears.

It is only a minority of those treated with cortisone who develop this syndrome, for it is related to the dosage of the drug as well as the duration of use. However anyone on steroids must be weaned off them with extreme care, as their own adrenal cortex will be suppressed from lack of ACTH, so they are totally dependent on an external supply to protect them from going into 'acute adrenal failure' or 'Addisonian crisis'.

Addison's disease is the opposite condition to Cushings, for here the body has effectively run out of hydrocortisone, which is required for protection against stress. It may arise from destruction of the adrenal cortex by tumour, including metastatic cancers, from TB, or more commonly from an autoimmune process similar to that of Hashimoto's disease, and indeed the two sometimes coincide. The symptoms are essentially the reverse of those of hyperadrenalism – weakness, low blood pressure, loss of weight and hypoglycaemia leading eventually to coma. There is often a darkening of the skin with pigmentation especially of the nipples and the inside of the cheeks if the disease has been gradually progressing for a long time.

Diabetes Mellitus

The pancreas has already featured in the digestive disorders, but here we are interested in the more common consequence of pancreatic dysfunction, diabetes mellitus (not to be confused with diabetes insipidus, an entirely unrelated disorder). Diabetes mellitus (Gr. mellis = sweet) occurs as a result of diminution or absence of insulin supplied by the beta cells of the Islets of Langerhans. Complete atrophy of the cells is more likely to occur in children and adolescents, leading suddenly to what is known as *juvenile-onset diabetes.*

In the middle-aged and elderly, diabetes usually results from insufficient insulin for the amount of tissue it has to supply, so there is often a degree of obesity and the condition is known as *maturity-onset diabetes.* Obviously the former cases will require insulin, which must be taken in the form of an injection as it is rapidly destroyed by the secretions of the stomach, whereas the latter type are usually able to stabilise their blood sugar on diet alone or with the addition of drugs to stimulate the beta cells.

The cause of the destruction of the beta-cells is in the vast majority of cases completely unknown, but destruction by an autoimmune process is speculated. In a very small percentage of cases the pancreas is damaged by a tumour or pancreatitis. Certainly there is an increased risk of the condition among the relatives of those who suffer from it, and among those of Jewish extraction, indicating a genetic component in the aetiology.

The symptomatology of the types is rather different. Juvenile-onset diabetics are seen less frequently but the onset is fairly rapid over a few weeks, and is often precipitated by an illness or infection. There will be a feeling of weakness and poor appetite as glucose is unable to enter the cells and builds up in the blood leading to *hyperglycaemia.* Once it reaches a certain level it can no longer be retained by the kidney and overflows into the urine as *glycosuria,* taking with it considerable quantities of water to carry it, so *polyuria* and *nocturia* develop. To compensate for this the patient becomes *thirsty* and drinks more, often craving sweet things. The glycosuria may lead to *infections* developing such as cystitis, balanitis and pruritus vulvae, while the increase in glucose in the aqueous humour of the eye alters the vision to cause blurring and difficulty focussing.

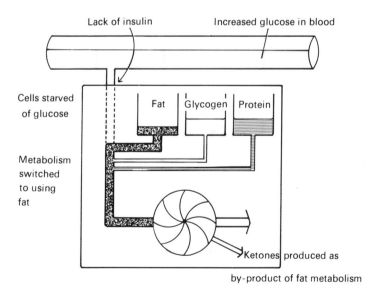

Fig. 16.1   *Cellular metabolism of glucose in A. normal and B. diabetic*

Because insulin facilitates the entry of glucose into the cells, its disappearance means that other arrangements have to be made to supply the cells with energy, and this comes in the form of fat which is taken from the body stores (see figure 16.1). The patient therefore starts to lose weight and when the fat is used to create energy it produces large quantities of acidic substances called *ketones* which are toxic to the body and so are rapidly excreted by both the lungs and the kidney (*ketonuria*). By the time such a situation has been reached the patient is usually *dehydrated* from the glycosuria and ketonuria, and has become somewhat stuporose from the build-up of acids in the blood, or even become unconscious in *diabetic coma*. In order to rid the body of the ketones more rapidly, the respiratory centre is stimulated to breathe more deeply and quickly – *air hunger* or 'Kussmaul's breathing' – and acetone can be smelt on the breath. If insulin and intravenous fluids are not received the patient's condition is likely to deteriorate and before the advent of insulin was invariably fatal.

In maturity-onset diabetics such a dramatic turn of events is seldom seen as some insulin is present, and indeed many patients have no symptoms at all and their diabetes is only discovered on a routine urinalysis. So why does it matter whether or not the condition is discovered? The answer is that over a number of years complications set in which can be greatly reduced if treatment is started early, and some maturity-onset diabetics can present initially with symptoms of the complications. These include leg cramps, ulcers, infections, poor vision, tingling in the hands and feet and vague complaints such as apathy or tiredness.

Complications of Diabetes. Because diabetes is a condition which continues for the duration of a patient's life there is an accumulation of side-effects which develop with time, although these can be minimized with effective control of the blood sugar. These are:

—*Atherosclerosis*, which occurs much more frequently because of the simultaneous disruption of fat metabolism in diabetics and leads to intermittent claudication, gangrene and ulcers in the feet, as well as heart attacks, strokes and hypertension.

—*Infections* are especially common in diabetics. As well as those of the urinary tract mentioned, some diabetics are troubled with persistant skin infections, vaginitis and boils, while TB is also more likely to occur.

—*Peripheral neuropathy* is a disorder or the peripheral nerves caused by damage to their blood supply by the diabetes. The sensory nerves are most often affected with tingling (paraesthesiae) and numbness of the arms and legs, later followed by weakness and paralysis. If the autonomic nerves are affected then failure of erection and impotence may result, or persistant diarrhoea.

—*Renal disease.* A particular kind of lesion occurs in the glomerular capillaries of many diabetics leading to thickening and ultimately chronic renal failure and uraemia. This complication is usually announced by the appearance in the urine of persistant proteinuria, but may take many years before complete failure ensues.

—*Retinopathy.* This is the commonest complication of young diabetics and leads to blindness in a small proportion. The retinal capillaries start to disintegrate and leak blood into the vitreous which causes scarring and distortion. As a result of the stimulus new capillaries may start to grow out into the vitreous and further obliterate vision, and it is these which are destroyed with the aid of a laser to preserve vision. As well as retinopathy, cataracts are slightly more common in diabetics.

Treatment of Diabetes.

This is along the three lines already mentioned – insulin, diet and what are called 'oral hypoglycaemic' drugs.

Insulin is usually necessary for the juvenile-onset type who are sometimes known as *insulin dependent* diabetics, and this is usually injected once or twice a day just before a meal. Different types of insulin are released at different rates into the blood, so by mixing them in a single morning dose it is possible to supply the body continually throughout the next 24 hours with only minor fluctuations in the blood level. This does, of course, depend on a very steady and regular intake of food, and if meals are missed then problems can arise. Some diabetics, however, are variable in their response, so their blood sugar level oscillates wildly up and down no matter how hard they try to regulate their diet, and they are sometimes termed *brittle diabetics*. This happens particularly during pregnancy in some women. If the blood glucose descends below a certain level they develop the symptoms of *hypoglycaemia* – sweating, weakness, palpitations, tremor and eventually confusion and coma, and in a minority such events may happen with dramatic suddenness, and are known as *insulin comas*. Such episodes are more likely if a meal is missed, so diabetics should carry an emergency supply of glucose tablets. One problem which sometimes occurs in the treatment of diabetics is to decide whether their unconsciousness is due to diabetic or insulin coma, for the treatment is different and to give too much insulin is very dangerous, so if there is doubt it is better to give glucose.

Diet is necessary for all diabetics, both in order to lose weight so as to conserve the existing supplies of insulin, and in order to balance the quantity of injected insulin. In most maturity-onset diabetics diet alone will clear the urine of glucose, but sometimes the assistance of drugs which act on the pancreas is needed. About one third of diabetics take them but they may require the addition of insulin in the event of an acute illness such as influenza.

17

Brain: Disorders of Communication

It is usual to divide the nervous system into the central part, consisting of the brain and spinal cord, and the peripheral nervous system, the spinal, cranial and autonomic nerves. In practice this neat division is not followed exactly by neurological diseases, but is attempted here nonetheless in order to simplify an otherwise extensive discussion, and peripheral nerve disorders are dealt with in the next chapter.

Strokes

The term aptly describes a condition of the brain characterised by its abrupt onset and widespread effects. Strokes were previously referred to as *apoplexy*, and the current medical term of *cerebro-vascular accident* or CVA indicates the underlying pathological basis of a vascular disorder. Because the brain is especially vulnerable to oxygen lack, it is well supplied by four major arteries which link together at the base to form the Circle of Willis, enabling blood flow to be restored in the event of one artery failing. From this circle a number of branches penetrate the brain, and these are particularly liable to *atherosclerosis* and its attendant complications of *haemorrhage, embolism* and *thrombosis*. Depending on the site chosen, the symptoms may cover a wide range from visual disturbance and dizziness to paralysis and anaesthesia, and the different types of underlying pathology will reflect the speed of onset and progress of the symptoms.

Who, then is at risk from strokes? By and large strokes occur more in women than in men and particularly those with *hypertension* or *diabetes* or in fact any condition leading to atherosclerosis including smoking and familial hypercholeste-rolaemia. The incidence in the over 65s is relatively high, about one in 500, and this makes it the commonest cause of death after coronary heart disease and cancer. However one person in three who gets a stroke will recover more or less completely in time, so the prognosis is by no means uniformly poor. Occasionally young people are at risk from a CVA because they develop malignant hypertension.

In the elderly the underlying pathology is more often a thrombosis and the symptoms will usually come on over a few hours or days, sometimes occurring at night when the circulation is most sluggish. There is often weakness of a limb or both limbs on one side of the body, numbness or dysphasia (difficulty speaking) and perhaps even loss of consciousness, at least for a while.

If the cause is an embolus, this will often arise in an area of atherosclerosis which may be distant from the brain, or in the wall of the heart following an infarction (mural thrombus), but may be quickly broken up by the flow of blood, so the symptoms are only transient, the episode being referred to as a *transient ischaemic attack* (TIA). Such attacks may involve the visual cortex and lead to the symptom of *amaurosis* (temporary blindness) with the sense of a curtain being drawn across the visual field, or there may be a transient *hemiplegia* (weakness of one half of the body) lasting minutes or hours and then recovering. A TIA is often a warning that a major stroke is about to happen within a few months.

Occasionally elderly people develop a more generalised form of cerebrovascular atherosclerosis which leads to widespread atrophy and *senile dementia*, of which it is one cause. The symptoms here take the form of confusion, intellectual deterioration, loss of memory and interest and emotional instability.

Subarachnoid Haemorrhage

Just as haemorrhage can occur within the brain tissue in the form of intracerebral haemorrhage mentioned above, so it may occur under or between the coverings of the brain, the meninges, and is known variously as subarachnoid, subdural or extradural depending on the exact location.

Of these the commonest is a *subarachnoid haemorrhage*, that is leakage of blood into the space beneath the arachnoid layer normally occupied by the CSF, and this usually derives from the rupture of a congenital defect of the Circle of Willis which takes

Skull

Dura

Intracerebral haemorrhage

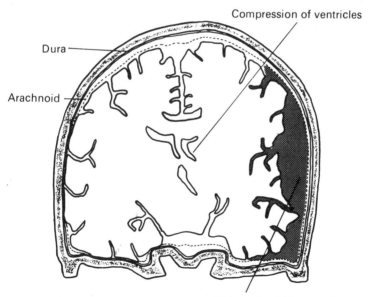

Compression of ventricles

Dura

Arachnoid

Subarachnoid haemorrhage

Fig. 17.1 *Cross section of brain to show A. Intracerebral haemorrhage (stroke), and B. subarachnoid haemorrhage* the form of a *berry aneurysm*. The composer Mendelssohn died at the age of 38 from just such a cause, as did his sister, father and grandfather, and it is notable that he complained of severe headaches for months before he succumbed, when the aneurysm was slowly leaking. This is the main symptom and is described as a stiffness in the neck, sometimes coming on very suddenly and accompanied by photophobia, nausea, dizziness and even loss of consciousness. The young and middle-aged are particularly affected, more often women, and those with hypertension are especially susceptible. If there is doubt about the diagnosis then examination of the CSF by lumbar puncture will show bloodstained fluid, and if necessary an Xray of the vessels of the brain incorporating contrast medium (angiogram) will show the exact position of the leak, which may require an operation to tie it off.

Subdural haemorrhage develops, as the name suggests, beneath the dura and is seen mostly in the very young and the elderly. It is liable to occur in babies born prematurely and in whom the skull bones are still soft and allow damage to the veins which cross the subdural space. Such infants may become permanently brain-damaged by such a bleed, and this is one reason for the application of forceps to protect the head from compression during birth. In the elderly this condition may follow a mild blow to the head, sometimes taking many weeks to manifest fully as the slow leakage of blood compresses the brain tissue and leads to gradual drowsiness, weakness, confusion and headaches. An operation to remove the collecting clot of blood may be needed.

Extradural haemorrhage arises from a head injury which ruptures the outermost vessels and causes a substantial bleed, resulting in symptoms soon after the injury. These will vary with the severity of the trauma, the most mild being a severe headache, nausea and vomiting, but sometimes progressing to loss of consciousness or deep coma.

Infections

The central nervous system is well insulated from most infectious processes by the possession of a barrier in the form of the meninges, and the only route in is via the bloodstream unless the skull is fractured or infected. In the event of an infection occurring it is more likely to involve the coverings of the brain as meningitis than the brain tissue itself when it takes the form of encephalitis.

Meningitis may be of bacterial or viral origin, and most of the epidemics are associated with the *meningococcus* organism which is spread by droplet infection from throat to throat and thence to the meninges. Periodically epidemics are liable to break out, in which case all age groups may be affected although the most at risk from the illness are young babies, in whom the diagnosis is most difficult. This is due to the fact that many of the symptoms of meningitis are non-specific. Instead of the classic *headache, photophobia* and *neck stiffness* seen in adults, there may be only pyrexia, vomiting and sometimes febrile convulsions which are common to other disorders, and the only certain way to establish the diagnosis is to perform a lumbar puncture. If treatment is not forthcoming then the disease progresses to meningeal irritability and neck stiffness, and sometimes a rash of pink spots on the trunk. The fontanelle on the skull will begin to bulge and eventually the spine will arch in a spasm (opisthotonous) owing to extension of the inflammation downwards. Now rarely seen in this country, but still common in the third world, is tuberculous meningitis which derives from a focus elsewhere in the body spreading via the blood into the meninges.

Encephalitis is almost invariably a viral infection and may accompany many of the more common viral illnesses such as influenza, mumps and glandular fever, in which it is the cause of the severe headache. Occasionally, however, the condition progresses to other symptoms – fits, drowsiness, paralysis or coma, and may lead to lasting damage. Some cases of Parkinsonism are attributable to previous attack by encephalitis virus.

An unusual and somewhat mysterious type of encephalitis is thought to arise as a result of infection by the Coxsackie virus and takes the form of extreme muscular fatigue and emotional lethargy so has been given the name 'post-viral fatigue syndrome' or *myalgic encephalitis*. The person suffers greatly from exhaustion which is liable to be dismissed as neurosis or hysteria (it was once known as the Royal Free Disease after an outbreak at that hospital), and this may last for many years before finally 'burning out', leaving a weakened immune system susceptible to infections especially by Candida.

Cerebral abscess is a type of infection not often seen, caused by the local spread of infection through the skull from a focus usually in the middle ear or sinuses, or sometimes from a more distant blood-borne site. As the abscess expands it causes syptoms from pressure, such as headache, nausea and vomiting, but is also accompanied by fever and later paralysis or weakness.

Headache

This extremely common symptom is almost always caused by changes in the vessels or tension in the muscles rather than intracerebral pathology, but it is obviously important to exclude the latter. So-called *tension headaches* are thought to occur from contraction of the muscles of the neck (from withdrawal and fear) or of the scalp and around the eyes (grief and sadness). They are characterised by increasing as the day wears on, but are alleviated usually by sleep.

Migraine is another very common form, but here the term specifically indicates a headache caused by alteration of the vessels, either from hormonal changes as occurs around the period, from the contraceptive pill or following the consumption of certain foods, particularly milk, eggs, cheese, chocolate, oranges, tomatoes, alcohol and some additives such as tartrazine.

The symptoms of migraine are only too well known to those who suffer from them, and attacks usually start with distorted vision and flashing lights, coloured zig-zag lines across the field of vision (*fortification spectra* or 'teichopsia'), *difficulty focussing* and *photophobia*. These are caused by an initial contraction of vessels in the visual cortex, which later expand to cause the characteristic throbbing, bursting sensation lasting sometimes for hours. If the attack is severe, there may also be tingling and numbness, often around the mouth, but sometimes involving a limb and even causing temporary paralysis. The headache usually starts on one side of the head (*hemicrania*) and is accompanied by nausea, vomiting and sometimes diarrhoea.

Certain variations of classical migraine occur, including *cluster headaches* which are typically severe, neuralgic pains situated around the eye and occurring in clusters every few weeks or months, then disappearing completely in between. They are often accompanied by redness and watering of the eye and perhaps a nasal discharge also. Some children develop recurrent abdominal pain and vomiting which has a certain similarity to migraine and is therefore sometimes known as *abdominal migraine*. Certainly there is a higher than average incidence of migrainous headaches in later life.

Orthodox treatment for migraine uses drugs containing ergotamine, a drug which constricts the vessels and thus counteracts the dilatation which causes the headache, sometimes with the addition of an antiemetic. These drugs are sometimes given in the form of suppositories for speed of action, but an excessive amount will lead to Raynaud's phenomenon (see chapter 10).

Raised intracranial pressure is a term used to describe a situation resulting from a variety of causes such as *malignant hypertension, brain tumour* and *abscess,* and which leads to a characteristic occipital pain which is worst on rising in the morning but tends to improve with upright posture as the day progresses. It is a persistant pain, made worse by any kind of straining, bending or coughing which increase the pressure of the CSF, and often accompanied by sudden vomiting without nausea owing to direct stimulation of the vomiting centre. There may also be accompanying visual disturbance or diplopia with dizziness from pressure on sensitive areas, and epileptic fits may occur in the case of intracranial tumours. A similar type of pain caused by meningeal irritation is seen in meningitis as already mentioned, and also following a lumbar puncture due to the sudden lowering of the pressure of the cerebrospinal fluid.

Not all headaches are a result of meningeal or vascular stimulation, and the possibility of referred pain in the head from a neighbouring structure must be born in mind, particularly the eyes, sinuses, cranial nerves and cervical spine. *Glaucoma* is an uncommon but elusive pain , being transmitted to the head, face or even abdomen. *Sinusitis* will mostly exhibit tenderness of the relevant area, while neuralgia of the cranial nerves is characteristic. *Trigeminal neuralgia* is the usual culprit, less often the glossopharyngeal nerve, and the pain is sudden, severe and lancinating, often being stimulated by chewing or touching the affected part, and radiating over the area supplied by the lower parts of the trigeminal nerve. *Tic douloureux* is the alternative name, and it is a condition of elderly people unless it represents an early symptom of multiple sclerosis which it may rarely do in the young. Pain in the upper division of the nerve is usually the first evidence of herpes zoster or *shingles* (q.v.) as this is its preferred site.

Epilepsy

Strictly speaking epilepsy is a symptom rather than a disease, albeit often quite a dramatic one, but in the majority of cases there is no observable pathology in the nervous tissues involved and so the cause remains a mystery. Normally neurones transmit nerve impulses in an orderly fashion, but in epileptics they discharge simultaneously and chaotically, leading to behaviour described as a fit, the exact nature of which depends on the location of the discharge (Gr. epilepto = to seize hold). About 1 person in 200 suffers from some form of epilepsy, and there is a tendency for it to run in families, being more common in children because of their more easily stimulated nervous systems, especially in the event of a high fever. Epilepsy arising for the first time in an adult is always a rather suspicious sign that some serious underlying condition such as a tumour or abscess has arisen.

There are three main types of epilepsy – grand mal, petit mal and temporal lobe epilepsy. Each of these has its own peculiarities of altered consciousness as described below, and will also be reflected in a typical abnormality of the brain wave pattern shown on the electroencephalogram (EEG).

Grand mal epilepsy is a form of generalised but temporary convulsion which may, however, be repeated, sometimes several times a day. The usual stages are four in number:

—*The aura*, during which the epileptic will have a premonition that an attack is about to happen, and which is felt either as a change in mood some days before, or perhaps as a definite sensation only a few seconds or minutes prior to the attack. It could be a smell, a sound or even a sense of deja vu, of having been here before, but is the same on each occasion.

—*The tonic phase* is when unconsciousness suddenly occurs and the person falls to the ground, sometimes injuring themselves, and remains rigid for a few moments without breathing, so becomes slightly blue.

—*The clonic phase* then follows, which consists of jerking movements (clonus) of the whole body, when the tongue may be bitten or urine voided and there is often frothing at the mouth. This usually passes into the last or

—*The relaxation phase*, when a stuporose, sleepy state supervenes for a variable time and then a gradual return to full consciousness happens.

If there is a delay in coming out of the clonic phase and the patient remains continually twitching, a situation sometimes seen in drug withdrawal or head injuries, this is termed *status epilepticus* (c.f. status asthmaticus) and leads to a state of permanent neural damage and possible fatality unless adequately treated.

Petit mal is a milder and more localised type of lapse of lucidity seen mostly in children who generally outgrow it (although it may rarely become grand mal later). There is a brief moment of 'absence' for a few seconds, during which the child is completely unaware of what is taking place around them and does not respond to questions. Sometimes there is a twitch of the arm or head, but they usually continue in what they were doing without pause.

Temporal lobe epilepsy is, as the name suggests, localised in the temporal lobe where memory and some sensations are coordinated. There is thus a disturbance in the content of consciousness rather than of consciousness itself, leading to hallucinations of hearing, taste or sight, or to dream-like states when automatic acts or untypical behaviour is exhibited, later completely forgotten.

Patients suffering from the above forms of epilepsy are not permitted to drive if they have had daytime fits within the previous two years, but may still qualify if they are restricted to nocturnal attacks.

Febrile convulsions are a very common type of fit seen in children up to the age of five when in the throes of a feverish illness. They represent a sudden increase in the susceptibility of the brain to excitation, and there is often a history of similar attacks in the family. The parents can be reassured that they do not lead to persistant epilepsy later and that the attacks are unlikely to be harmful unless they become continuous. Nevertheless it is important to exclude an underlying condition, especially meningitis.

Multiple Sclerosis

The nerve fibres of the brain and spinal cord are enclosed within a white sheath made of a fatty substance called myelin, and without the presence of this they are unable to conduct impulses. Multiple or disseminated sclerosis is a disease characterised by *demyelination* of the nerves in a more or less random manner, so that its symptoms are correspondingly variable and diagnosis made difficult. As the areas of demyelination heal there is corresponding atrophy or sclerosis of the nerves worst affected, but others regain their function, so that the disease proceeds in a stepwise fashion with acute episodes followed by partial recovery, but is usually progressive. The overall duration of the disease is very variable and depends to a large extent on which functions of the body are mainly affected, but many patients live for 30 years or more from the time of diagnosis.

The aetiology is unknown, although various theories abound. One current one is that the body is earlier sensitised by being infected by a virus which causes damage to the myelin at a much later stage. Whatever the cause MS is a condition of temperate countries and is much less common in the tropics, in fact the incidence increases corresponding to the distance from the equator. Young or middle aged adults are the usual victims, which number 1 in 2000 of the population in this country, and women are slightly more at risk than men.

The initial symptoms are variable, but those most commonly seen are:

—transient tingling or numbness in an area of the body, lasting a few days and then clearing up. A whole limb or only a small area may be affected, and may be followed by increased sensitivity for a while.

—weakness of a hand or foot causing unaccustomed clumsiness or a tendency to trip easily. At times this will start after hard excercise or a hot bath.

—unsteadiness or staggering (*ataxia*) of the whole body, due to involvement of the cerebellum.

—blurred vision due to involvement of the optic nerve (*optic* or *retrobulbar neuritis*).

—double vision due to damage to the nerves supplying the extrinsic muscles of the eye.

—slurred speech (*dysarthria*).

The usual story is for the earlier symptoms to partly or completely clear after a week or two, sometimes never to return but more often to reoccur months later in similar form, with additional features. These may include:

—difficulty voiding urine (retention) or incontinence of urine.

—shooting pains down the back.

—painful spasms in the limbs.

—emotional changes, either depression or more often a degree of euphoria.

The main long-term problems for MS sufferers are the lack of control of the bladder which leads to urinary infections, the difficulty with walking which may mean using a wheelchair and eventually total paralysis, death being due to the chest infections resulting from immobility.

Parkinson's Disease

In 1817 Dr Parkinson described a condition commonly seen in the elderly which was characterised by rigidity and tremor and to which he gave the name *paralysis agitans* or the 'shaking palsy'. It is one of the most frequently met neurological conditions, seen in about 1 in 400 of the population over the age of 65, and caused by a decrease in the amount of the neurotransmitter *dopamine* found in the *basal ganglia*, the area of the brain responsible for the coordination of movement. Most of the cases are due to either atherosclerosis or unknown degenerative changes, but very occasionally in younger individuals the disorder is a result of poisoning or encephalitis. A very similar condition results as a side-effect of drug treatment for schizophrenia.

The clinical features of the disorder fall into two main categories, *tremor* and *rigidity*. The tremor is very typical and takes the form of a slow, coarse, regular shaking of the fingers and limbs, producing a characteristic 'pill-rolling' movement of the thumb and forefinger. This disappears during voluntary movement and comes back at rest so is known as a *resting tremor*.

However, tremor is the least disabling aspect , what is more of a problem is the stiffness and poverty of movement which may develop, and which causes difficulty in initiating activities such as walking, although once started a repetetive action can be maintained though it is done stiffly and awkwardly. This rigidness, as well as being painful, causes difficulty with things like fastening buttons and shoelaces, writing, swinging the arms when walking and even speaking smoothly and clearly. There is a slowing of all movements and the facial expression becomes stiff and masklike, the eyes seldom blink and the gait becomes a shuffle with frequent falls. Other features sometimes seen are excessive salivation, tiredness and depression.

To distinguish Parkinsonism from other types of tremor is usually not difficult. The tremors of anxiety and hyper-thyroidism are more rapid, and so-called 'senile tremor' is continuous and does not fluctuate, being more of a kind of 'ditheriness'. Tremor arising from cerebellar disorders, while also causing ataxia, becomes worse on voluntary movement rather than improving (*intentional tremor*). When the arm or leg of someone with Parkinsonism is moved passively the combination of tremor and stiffness causes the characteristic 'cogwheel phenomenon', but sometimes tremor is absent and the rigidness is then described as 'lead pipe rigidity' as the limb suddenly 'gives' once the rigidity is overcome.

Treatment of Parkinsonism depends on replacing the missing dopamine by giving L–dopa in tablet form, which improves the rigidity but has a less marked effect on the tremor. Unfortunately the drugs have side-effects in the form of nausea and vomiting, and sometimes cardiac arrhythmias.

18

Nerve: Disorders of Feeling and Movement

Interruption, pressure or damage to the peripheral nerves may be the cause of pain or weakness in parts of the body supplied by them, and although there is considerable overlap with the nerves of the central nervous system the distinction is nevertheless useful. In general, if the reflex arc is intact as judged by the tendon reflexes, then it is unlikely that the peripheral nerves are involved, and this is one of the main uses of the test.

Entrapment Syndromes

There are many places in the body where nerves run in restricted spaces and are thus liable to compression from neighbouring structures such as bones, ligaments or fibrous tissue. These 'entrapment syndromes' as they are termed are very common, and two of them, *sciatica* and *carpal tunnel syndrome*, have already been described.

Brachial neuralgia is the name given to the pains which develop in the arm if the nerve is stretched by carrying heavy weights or compressed by one of the discs in the cervical vertebrae which is misplaced. The initial symptoms are usually *paraesthesiae* (pins and needles) running down the arm, followed by shooting pains and weakness of the muscles in the hands with a tendency to drop things. The pains may be present when the neck is flexed or the head turned, and there will often be tenderness over the affected disc.

On occasions a similar pain is felt down the front of the thigh in overweight individuals after they have been walking or standing for a while. This is due to compression of the lateral cutaneous nerve of the thigh where it runs under the inguinal ligament, and goes by the name of 'meralgia paraesthetica'.

Another place in the leg where nerves are liable to entrapment is immediately below the head of the fibula, either after an injury or in those who kneel crosslegged with one leg tucked underneath them. There is numbness of the upper part of the foot or even weakness of dorsiflexion of the ankle and 'foot drop'.

Peripheral Neuropathy

The peripheral nerves are also liable to more diffuse disease, arising either from interference to the blood vessels which supply them, or from direct poisoning by toxins or drugs, or in some instances to allergy. Usually the neuropathy is secondary to an established condition such as diabetes mellitus, alcoholism or vitamin deficiency, in which case it comes on gradually as 'neuralgic' pains in the limbs with weakness, and is sometimes referred to as 'polyneuritis'. Sometimes only a single nerve is involved and then a 'mononeuritis' is the result, most commonly seen in diabetics.

One somewhat notorious type of polyneuritis is that known as *Guillain-Barre syndrome* which occasionally follows immunisation or viral infections such as glandular fever, measles and herpes infections. A widespread outbreak in the USA followed the mass immunisation programme against influenza in 1976. The symptoms arrive rapidly, usually in the space of a few hours, with tingling and numbness in the arms and legs which spreads up the limbs to the trunk. The muscles weaken and become quite tender, and if the attack is severe then assisted respiration may be required for the duration of the acute phase, although the patient remains fully conscious as the higher centres are not involved. After several weeks the slow recovery begins and may take six months or more before completed, but there is seldom any residual disability. The most likely cause of this rather strange affliction is an allergic reaction by the body, possibly of an autoimmune variety.

Spina Bifida

As the embryo develops in the first few weeks of life, the vertebrae and spinal cord are formed by an infolding of the outermost layer of tissues which unite together to become the 'neural tube'. In the case of spina bifida there is a *neural tube defect* (NTD) to a variable degree when the tissues fail to join, so either just the vertebrae remain divided ('spina bifida occulta'), or the whole of the spinal cord lies exposed, covered only by a thin membrane, and the nerves themselves are atrophied.

About one baby in every 700 is born with a degree of spina bifida sufficient to affect function, and recently it has been possible to diagnose the condition before birth with accuracy by sampling the amniotic fluid and examining the protein secreted by the exposed tube, *alpha foetoprotein.* Not only is this present in large quantities in the amniotic sac, but some circulates in the mother's blood and a fair estimation of the presence of NTD may be made from this. The lumbo-sacral region is the area most likely to be affected, and about one person in six has some

Normal development

Occult spina bifida (symptomless)   Severe spina bifida

Fig. 18.1   *Section through vertebrae showing position of spinal cord in neural tube defects* evidence of a slight failure of the vertebrae to fuse, shown by a small dimple with a tuft of hair in it at the base of the spine.

Many possible causes have been proposed to account for spina bifida, ranging from measles to the consumption of green potatoes in pregnancy, but none have been substantiated even after extensive investigation. Recent trials, however, have indicated that vitamin deficiency shortly before and during pregnancy may be a factor, and supplements are recommended for the first eight weeks. Mothers who take the antiepileptic drug Epilim may also be at an increased risk.

If a child is born with severe spina bifida it is the legs and bladder which are most affected, with weakness and lack of sphincter control in later life, leading to either retention or incontinence and frequent urinary infections. There may be impaired sensation to the legs and hence damage to the skin and subsequent ulceration. Men are liable to suffer from impotence because of the involvement of the nerves of erection, and this should be considered as a possible cause when investigating this condition.

If the spina bifida at birth is large and exposed to the air, then a decision must be made within a day or so as to whether to operate and close it, for otherwise infection to the cord and meningitis is a real risk. Many babies with severe NTD have an associated *hydrocephalus* on account of a blockage to the aqueduct leading out of the ventricles of the brain.

Bell's Palsy

This is a condition of the seventh cranial nerve, the one which supplies the muscles of facial expression and taste. The nerve happens to run within a narrow bony canal at the point where it exits from the middle ear, and sometimes swells if the ear is exposed to a draught for a long period, or following an ear infection. Because it is unable to expand the oedema will prevent impulses passing down to the face which consequently becomes paralysed on one side. Thus the brow droops down and the person is unable to close their eye which rolls up under the lid, nor can they frown or smile. The mouth sags and may cause slight dribbling, and tears will flow from the weakened eyelids. Sometimes there will be some loss of taste, and noises may be heard very intensely as the stapedius muscle in the ear, which normally dampens loud sounds, is put out of action. Over half of those with Bell's palsy recover fully in 6 weeks or so and most of the remainder are left with only a minor disability.

Mouth droops   Unable to close eye

Fig. 18.2   *Right sided Bell's palsy A. with face relaxed, and B. on grimacing*

19

Eye: Disorders of Vision

Vision is the sense which we can project over the furthest distance, literally beyond the stars, by making use of certain frequencies of electromagnetic radiation we call light. With this sense we can perceive danger at a much greater distance than sound or touch, but it has two drawbacks – the source must be in a direct line of vision, and there must be sufficient light reflected off the source which is often not the case at night. Because light waves do not travel round corners, our eyes must therefore be freely mobile, and the best solution lies in a ball and socket arrangement. In order to maintain the spherical shape of the globe, the eyeball must be pressurised from within by fluid, and the pressure contained by a strong outer coat – the sclera (Gr = hard). This coat withstands trauma and infection well, so this is generally confined to the supporting tissues outside the eyeball.

In order to admit light the front of the sclera, the cornea, must be transparent, which means it is devoid of capillaries for the provision of nourishment and this is therefore provided by the tears from the lacrimal glands and by the aqueous humour in the anterior chamber. Moreover it must be well protected, a function of the very sensitive conjunctiva which covers it and of the lids which close reflexly in the event of threat. Finally, because the light reflected from an object is divergent, it must be concentrated by a focussing mechanism, the lens, on to the retina or we would see the world through a keyhole as it were. Of course the lens inverts the image on the screen, so we actually see the world upside down and leave it to our occipital cortex to right it again.

In such an immensely complex apparatus it is surprising that so few elements fail us, apart from the focussing mechanism for which we may need help. The most commonly occurring faults are in the lids and lacrimal apparatus, sometimes in the conjunctival membrane and less often on the cornea. Within the eyeball, apart from refractive errors, the usual problem is with aging changes in the lens – cataract, disorders of pressurisation – glaucoma and least often retinal and neural problems. Finally it must be remembered that the eyes operate as a pair and each looks at an object from a slightly different angle. Failure to do this results in a squint (strabismus), most frequently seen in children.

Lacrimal Problems

These are first seen in the time immediately following birth in babies suffering from *sticky eye*, caused by a narrowing of the tear duct where it crosses the bone below the eye. Quite often the duct is immature and does not fully develop for several months, during which time the tears well up and overflow down the cheeks. During the night they form a stagnant pool which evaporates and thickens, so that on waking the eyelids are encrusted and stuck together, sometimes slightly infected. Treatment is to bathe away the crusts and then gently massage the lacrimal duct just below the inner corner of the eye. It is rare for the duct to need probing or syringing unless it fails to resolve spontaneously in 3-4 months. On occasions a similar condition may occur in adults, and lead to the symptom of *epiphora* – tears running down the cheeks.

Another cause of epiphora, usually in the elderly, is failure of the entrance of the lacrimal duct to approximate to the eyeball, because the tissues of the lower lid have either atrophied or been displaced by a Meibomian cyst (qv), giving the eye a red-rimmed appearance. This turning out of the lid is known as an *ectropion*, and the opposite condition or *entropion* leads to a similar result by allowing the lashes to abrade the conjunctiva.

At the inner aspect of the eye and just below it is the dilated lacrimal sac, a reservoir of tears which may be the focus for infection, leading to a swollen, inflamed lump called a 'dacryocystitis' (Gr. dacryos = tear). On pressure some pus can be seen oozing out of the punctum on the lower lid, and the eye will water.

Sjogren's syndrome is a condition of atrophy of the lacrimal glands leading to itching and grittiness and recurrent inflammation of the conjunctiva. It usually starts in middle-age, especially in women around the time of the menopause, and may be associated with rheumatoid arthritis or other connective tissue disorders. There is sometimes accompanying dryness of the salivary glands with dry mouth and soreness of the tongue.

A. Ectropion

B. Entropion

C. Meibomian cyst

D. Stye

Fig. 19.1   *Disorders of the eyelids*

The Lids

These are covered in front by a thin layer of skin and so are prone to a number of skin conditions, while behind is the conjunctival membrane which becomes inflamed in conjunctivitis (qv). At its centre the lid is stiffened by a plate of connective tissue – the tarsus, and it is here that tarsal cysts may arise from small glands within the tarsus known as Meibomian glands, whose function is to secrete sebaceous fluid which lubricates the lids.

Meibomian or *tarsal cysts* are not true cysts caused by blockage of a duct, but enlargement of the glandular tissue due to chronic irritation or infection and they tend to occur in crops. The gland becomes swollen and red and is also known as a 'chalazion' (Gr = a collection of rubble), being particularly prominent if the lid is everted and the back inspected, so the patient may complain of watering and irritation. Sometimes they become acutely inflamed and discharge pus, but can be differentiated from a stye (see below) by the position halfway up the lid.

A *stye* or 'hordeolum' (L. hordeum = barley) is an infection of the root of a lash, and thus is always found at the edge of the lid where it causes an inflamed swelling with a yellow head. Styes often contain staphylococci and there may be similar skin infections about such as boils or acne.

Blepharitis (Gr. blepharon = eyelid) is a chronic inflammation of the margin of the lids which are red, scaly and sometimes slightly swollen or even ulcerating. This condition is found in those predisposed to dandruff or seborrhoea and tends to lead to recurrent infections, including styes. The scales cling to the lashes and may be removed by bathing with 5% bicarbonate of soda in warm water. On occasions a more widespread blepharitis is a result of an allergy to cosmetics or eye drops.

Ptosis (Gr = falling) is the term given to drooping of the upper lid from paralysis of the muscles, most cases being congenital. In old age so-called 'senile ptosis' is simply due to sagging of the tissues which have become atrophied. Ptosis of sudden onset is more significant and if unilateral is then due either to paralysis of the third cranial nerve or to the sympathetic nerves in the neck (usually from a bronchial carcinoma). The latter leads to the triad of symptoms known as *Horner's syndrome*, a combination of ptosis, a sunken eye and a constricted pupil. Of course if the sympathetic nerves are stimulated the lids do the opposite and retract, and this is what typically occurs in hyperthyroidism.

Myaesthenia gravis is a disease characterised by a general weakness of the muscles, caused by an autoimmune disorder in which the chemical acetylcholine conducting the nerve impulse across the neuromuscular junction becomes depleted. The earliest feature is usually bilateral ptosis, and the lids drop progressively as the day wears on, followed by weakness of the other muscles of the body.

A skin condition which has a preference for the eyelids is *xanthelasma* (Gr. xanthos = yellow; elasma = plate) – thickened, yellow, waxy plaques on the upper or lower lids near the inner canthus and signifying excessive quantities of cholesterol in the blood, a tendency which is inherited or found in diabetics.

The Conjunctiva

This is the membrane which lines the back of the lids and also covers the front of the eyeball, so that when the eyes are closed it forms a complete sac containing tears. Not infrequently it becomes inflamed owing to exposure to dust, infection and allergens such as pollen, giving rise to various types of conjunctivitis. A very frequently met condition of the conjunctiva is a *subconjunctival haemorrhage*, which follows a spontaneous rupture of one of the capillaries and spreads across the white sclera, disfiguring the eye for a week or two but of no pathological significance unless repeated, when a haemorrhagic disorder should be considered.

Acute conjunctivitis is commonly due to bacterial infection, and if it is restricted to one eye this indicates that a foreign body is the probable cause. The sclera of the eye is pink or red and swollen, especially at the periphery, as is the tarsal conjunctiva, and epiphora may be prominent. Sometimes there is much oedema, a condition known as 'chemosis', and there may be a purulent discharge which sticks the lids together, along with some flecks of mucopus seen under the lids. The vision is essentially normal and the pupil is a regular shape and reacts to light.

If the condition occurs in a newborn baby then a gonorrhoeal cause must be considered – so-called 'ophthalmia neonatorum' – as this is a virulent infection which may lead to blindness if inadequately treated. It is, however, rare nowadays and most cases of neonatal conjunctivitis are associated with a chlamydial infection and called 'inclusion conjunctivitis' because of the way the chlamydia are included within the cells. The mother will usually be found to have a venereal infection. This form is occasionally caught by adults in swimming baths and seems to be becoming more common.

Trachoma is also a chlamydial conjunctivitis, rare in this country but on a world wide scale it is the most common cause of blindness. Cases are occasionally seen among immigrants from the middle and far east, appearing as chronic conjunctivitis.

Viral conjunctivitis occurs in schools and other communities as a local outbreak of 'pink eye', with slight fever and enlargement of the pre-auricular glands in front of the ear. It lasts only a few days and usually clears spontaneously.

Allergic conjunctivitis is not as a rule difficult to distinguish from an infective cause, and produces a clear, mucoid discharge with much itching. It assumes two forms, the first being that of hay fever and occurring in the summer months in conjunction with sneezing and catarrh. Less commonly a different, more localised allergy involving just the tarsal conjunctiva may occur, known as *vernal* or *spring catarrh* as it appears earlier in the year. The back of the lids assume a very swollen and rather alarming 'cobblestone' appearance, with large itchy swellings and characteristic ropy secretions.

A *pterygium* (Gr = wing) is sometimes seen on the nasal side of

Fig. 19.2A *Pterygium*

the eyeball, crossing the sclera as an opaque triangular encroachment. It is a degenerative change in the conjunctiva and mostly seen in dry, sunny countries where UV light is thought to be a causative factor. Unless it invades the cornea it is only really of cosmetic significance.

Fig. 19.2B *Arcus senilis*

The Cornea

The most frequently seen lesion on the cornea is the crescent or circle of lipid material, thickest at the top or bottom, termed an *arcus senilis*. It is separated from the margin of the cornea by a thin band of clear cornea and is a greyish colour. When seen in younger people it usually signifies an abnormally large quantity of lipid in the blood and is therefore associated with vascular pathology.

Inflammation of the cornea is termed *keratitis* and is usually associated with viruses as, with the exception of the gonococcus, bacteria can only invade the corneal epithelium if it is already damaged. It is for this reason that a corneal abrasion needs regular scrutiny to ensure that it does not become a corneal ulcer. The cornea is also damaged by drying as may occur in Sjogren's syndrome, trachoma and the exophthalmos of thyrotoxicosis if the lids fail to meet. Acne rosacea may lead to keratitis in some, and will improve as the skin condition resolves.

Herpes simplex keratitis is a form of cold sore occurring on the cornea, and takes the shape of tiny pinhead size dots or a ragged, branching ulcer known from its shape as *dendritic* (Gr. dendron=tree). Needless to say the condition is extremely painful, with photophobia and reddening of the sclera, along with some impairment of vision. Herpes zoster or *shingles* may also occur on the cornea if the ophthalmic nerve is affected and a blistering rash is seen on the forehead and side of the nose. This mostly affects elderly patients and is preceded and sometimes followed by a neuralgic pain along the course of the nerve. With both forms of keratitis, if a deep ulcer forms in the cornea then there is inflammation of the anterior chamber and the iris. Sterile pus gravitates to form a level at the bottom of the anterior chamber – a 'hypopyon', and the iris becomes swollen and engorged with blood – *acute iritis* (also called iridocyclitis).

The Uveal Tract

The diagram illustrates the proximity of the iris, ciliary body and choroid which are continuous with one another and together termed the 'uvea' or 'uveal tract' (Gr. uvea = hump-backed), and inflammation of the area is often termed *uveitis*. This has come to be virtually synonymous for 'iritis', 'iridocyclitis' and 'choroidi-tis' and the three expressions may be regarded as virtually interchangeable.

Since the uvea is enclosed within the eyeball, most cases of uveitis are not of infective origin but have an allergic or autoimmune basis. It seems that the cells of the iris are extremely sensitive to antigens and if one appears in the blood, as may happen in the chronic conditions mentioned below, the tissue reacts by inflaming and swelling, so uveitis is characterised by a deep, throbbing pain, redness at the edge of the cornea and constriction of the pupil. This is unfortunate as the congested iris is likely to become stuck to the lens immediately behind it by the exudate, and remain an irregular shape on account of these adhesions or 'synechiae' as they are termed (Gr. synechio = dance together). This is the reason for using atropine drops to dilate the pupil and prevent this.

The conditions mainly associated with uveitis are rheumatoid arthritis, sarcoidosis, ankylosing spondylitis, Reiter's syndrome, lupus erythematosis and Behcet's disease. The latter is an uncommon but very distressing and painful condition of unknown origin occurring mostly in young men who develop ulceration of the mouth and genitalia.

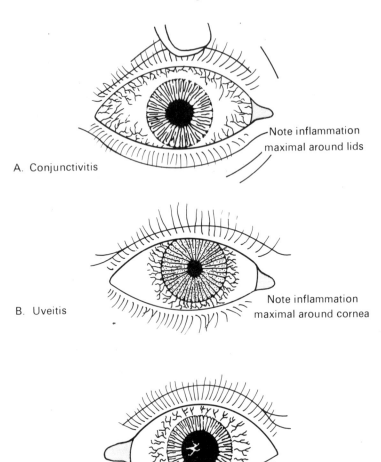

A. Conjunctivitis

Note inflammation maximal around lids

B. Uveitis

Note inflammation maximal around cornea

C. Dendritic ulcer

D. Subconjunctival haemorrhage

Fig. 19.3   *The common causes of a red eye*

Glaucoma

The pressure within the eye has to be finely balanced so that it is sufficient to maintain the roundness of the eyeball but not so great that it prevents blood from entering to nourish the retina. If it exceeds what is considered normal, about 20 mmHg as measured on the tonometer, then the retina will become ischaemic and we have the condition known as glaucoma. This develops because the outflow of the aqueous humour in the anterior chamber is obstructed, sometimes because the shape of the eye allows the lens to push the iris forward (*closed angle* or *acute glaucoma*) but often for no obvious reason (*open angle* or *chronic glaucoma*). In a few cases it may be secondary to uveitis which silts up the drainage channel with inflammatory debris.

Acute glaucoma occurs particularly in women in their 50s and 60s, and is due to narrowing of the angle of the anterior chamber by a long thin lens in a relatively small eye, so the patient is usually longsighted and wears thick glasses. Attacks come on suddenly after the pupil has dilated and closed the angle altogether, often at night, and are characterised by blurred vision, headaches and the appearance of coloured haloes around lights (Gr. glaucos = gleaming). These attacks recur and become more severe until there is intense congestion of the eye and serious visual damage. The orthodox treatment involves removing a small piece of the iris in each eye (peripheral iridectomy), to allow the humour to pass directly into the drainage channel.

Chronic glaucoma is more insidious in its manner of approach, and arises mostly in elderly people. It appears in eyes of all shapes and sizes and because its aetiology is completely unknown it is sometimes given the unfortunate name of 'simple glaucoma' although it is anything but! There may be a few slight headaches but in most patients the only sign is gradual onset of defects in the field of vision or *scotomas* (Gr = darkness) and therefore regular examination by an optician is desirable in this age group. If the retina is examined with an ophthalmoscope, a characteristic cup-shaped depression in the optic disc can be seen where the retina sags at its weakest point. Standard treatment is with pilocarpine or adrenaline drops to encourage the outflow, or beta-blocking drops to reduce the production of humour.

Canal where aqueous is absorbed   Canal obstructed

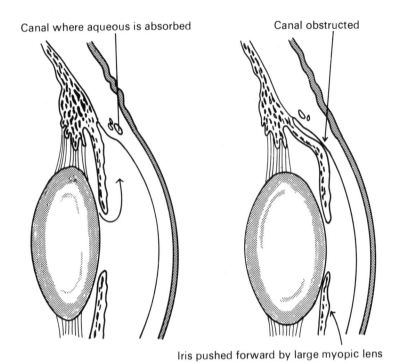

Iris pushed forward by large myopic lens

Fig. 19.4   *The circulation of aqueous humour in A. normal eye and B. acute glaucoma*

Cataract

The name derives from the Greek meaning 'accursed', and illustrates the dread in which patients hold this opacity of the lens, heralding as it does the last of the seven ages of man (and woman, for it occurs equally in both sexes). The age at which so-called 'senile cataract' starts is determined by genetic influence, as is the speed with which it progresses.

Cataracts are caused by the coagulation of the proteins of the lens with age, much as egg albumen coagulates on heating, and the opacities begin as wedge-shaped spokes around the edge of the lens with clear areas in between. These actually begin in early middle age, but we are not aware of them as that part of the lens is covered by the iris, and visual acuity is maximal through the centre of the lens. Eventually these wedges converge on the hub as it were and obscure central vision, but as well as spreading in this direction, the opacities spread from the inner layers of the lens to the outer (the lens is made of layers rather like an onion), and until they have reached the cortex the cataract is not 'ripe' and therefore technically more difficult to extract. Once it has become ripe it then starts to disintegrate and cause complications, so there is an optimal time at which to remove it and this is not always understood by patients. Recently the tendency has been to insert a small plastic lens in place of the natural one and use spectacles to change the focus. Sometimes this is not feasible and a contact lens or thick spectacles are used instead, but this has the disadvantage of magnifying everything and distorting vision.

The process of hydration and coagulation which leads to cataracts may be accelerated in certain circumstances, and *diabetes*, long-term *steroid therapy*, infra-red light and trauma are all liable to cause early cataracts, while congenital cataracts occur in rubella and Down's syndrome.

Retinal Disorders

The retina suffers like any other tissue from a variety of pathology – oedema, ischaemia, degeneration, detachment and even infection. However, because of its central role as a sensory receptor the retina responds by informing us rapidly with some form of impairment of vision at the least provocation.

Interference with the blood supply arises particularly in *diabetes* and *hypertension* and leads to both leakage from the vessels at the back of the 'fundus' of the eye, and to oedema of the retina (*papilloedema*), but this is only visible with an ophthalmoscope. Blindness in this country most commonly results from this so-called *diabetic retinopathy* which is a mixture of lack of nourishment, haemorrhage and exudation of fat, especially around the macula where damage is maximal. Furthermore, the ischaemic retina responds by promoting the growth of new vessels which only makes matters worse, and it is for the destruction of these that diabetics undergo laser treatment.

Senile macular degeneration is the name given to the atrophy of cells in the macula of the retina occurring in the elderly and leading to a central scotoma affecting the reading area of the eye so they have a severe impairment. A slightly similar condition affecting a much younger age group is *retinitis pigmentosa*, an inherited tendency to degeneration and pigmentation of the cones and even more the rods. This starts in childhood as night-blindness and leads to gradual tunnel vision and then complete blindness in middle age as the degeneration encroaches on the macula.

Retinal detachment is actually a split in the two layers of the retina, either due to a tear in the retina allowing vitreous fluid to seep through and raise the inner layer off its bed, as is seen in diabetes or a sudden blow to the eye; or else because the inner layer becomes attached to the vitreous which tugs at it and produces the standard retinal response – flashing lights. These are a warning that a detachment is impending, and can be differentiated from those of migraine by always being in exactly the same place. Once a detachment occurs, there is no pain but a curtain begins to fall across the field of vision as the retina comes away, and needs to be gently replaced and probably affixed with the judicious use of a coagulating laser.

Floaters or 'muscae volitantes' (L. musca = fly; volito = fluttering) are a different phenomenon altogether and consist of particles of collagen and other debris floating in the vitreous and observable by the subject against a light background and by the practitioner with an ophthalmoscope. Unless they suddenly appear in large numbers they are not pathological, but need to be carefully distinguished from the flashing lights mentioned above.

Squint

In normal development a newborn baby learns to focus its eyes on an object within a few weeks, and to do so it must have normal macular vision. During the learning process its eyes wander independently of one another, but soon learn that by working simultaneously as a pair they are able to judge the distance of an object, so binocular vision arrives. But what happens if one eye has greater difficulty in seeing than the other, either from a refractive error in the lens or from more serious pathology? This eye will then have difficulty focussing on the object, and even if it does the image will be in the wrong place and so double vision occurs which simply confuses the child. So the brain automatically suppresses the false image and the eye in question becomes lazy or *amblyopic* (Gr. amblyos = dim) and gradually ceases to function at all. Over the next few years the suppression continues until by the age of five or so it is permanent and the child is left with monocular vision. Moreover the amblyopic eye feels under no compunction to follow its colleague in the direction of its gaze and remains a social embarrassment to its owner who finds as he gets older that the wrong people (who he can't see) keep answering his questions.

Until the amblyopic eye finally gives up, the child may look at objects with either eye – 'alternate fixation' – but will not, as is sometimes believed, 'grow out of a squint'. In order to encourage the weaker eye to develop macular vision it is necessary to cover the good eye with a patch or even, if the image is falling far outside the macula, to correct the eye muscles surgically.

Sudden squints arising in adults may be due to damage to one of the nerves supplying the eye muscles, usually from diabetes, MS or occasionally a tumour or aneurysm compressing the nerve. These will cause diplopia for a few days until the false image is suppressed.

20

Ear: Disorders of Hearing and Balance

The ear is the organ of both hearing and balance, two of our most important senses, and is well protected by being sited deep within the temporal bone. This means that little is visible for examination, apart from the external part of the ear, and the functions of the middle and inner ear must be inferred from tests. Examination of the drum using an otoscope will be helped if the canal is straightened by gently pulling the ear upwards and backwards.

The External Ear

The pinna or auricle is a rudimentary funnel for sound which has little use in humans, and consists simply of cartilage covered in skin. The crease behind the auricle is a favorite site for sebaceous cysts to form, and the helix occasionally contains a tophus in gouty subjects, or is disfigured from repeated bruising in boxers with 'cauliflower ears'. Otherwise many of the problems of the external auditory canal are those of the skin which line it, and as this is a warm, moist locality eczema commonly features here and causes a chronic, itchy discharge and sometimes some small blisters. It may periodically become infected, especially if abraded by instruments used for cleaning wax from the ear, and then becomes painful, extremely so if a boil is present and will then be seen blocking the canal. *Otitis externa* is particularly likely to occur after swimming in dirty water when fungi can enter and set up a cheesy, white discharge, and if the subject is a child the possibility of a foreign body must be remembered as this is a favourite site for depositing small objects.

The Drum

The drum or *tympanic membrane* is an oval, semi-transparent membrane the size of a large pea in diameter, and set at the end of the 1″ long canal. It is normally a delicate pearly grey colour, and when inflamed goes an angry red and later a deep purple. This will happen if a middle ear infection occurs, or after swimming and diving or flying in pressurised aircraft, on account of the imbalance between the pressures on the different sides of the drum, known as *barotrauma*. During flight the aircraft is normally pressurised at a rather lower than normal pressure and some air leaves the Eustachian tube. On touchdown the pressure is then brought up to normal but if the air is unable to re-enter the tube because of catarrh then the drum will bulge inwards and severe pain may result along with deafness and vertigo, lasting several hours.

The Middle Ear

Otitis media is one of the commonest of childhood complaints and tends to occur whenever there is blockage of the Eustachian tube at the lower end on account of catarrh or enlarged adenoids. If a cold or other upper respiratory infection occurs then it will often progress upward into the middle ear and cause pain of a stabbing or throbbing nature. The secretions will become infected with staphylococci or streptococci and the drum will be seen to bulge under pressure from the pus and possibly eventually burst, which relieves the pain. Fortunately most perforations heal in a few weeks without complications once the pus is able to drain freely, and the slight deafness soon clears. If the drum does not perforate it will still heal fairly quickly and look scaly and a little like crazy paving.

Complications of otitis media are rare but need to be kept in mind as they are potentially serious, and usually involve extensions of the infection into other areas.

—*Mastoiditis* is one of the better known and occurs when infection travels into the hollow spaces of the mastoid bone behind the ear, which may happen quite suddenly. The bone becomes tender when pressed (and this should always be tested), there is swelling there and the auricle is pushed forward and sticks out. If a course of antibiotics has been aborted then this mastoiditis may be masked and build up slowly with continual pain in the ear.

—Extension of the infection upwards can very rarely penetrate the temporal bone and invade the meninges to cause meningitis or a *cerebral abscess*.

—The facial nerve runs across the Eustachian tube and so it is liable to damage here in the form of *Bell's palsy* (see Chapter 18).

—The inner ear may become involved which will announce itself by the vertigo and vomiting of *labyrinthitis*.

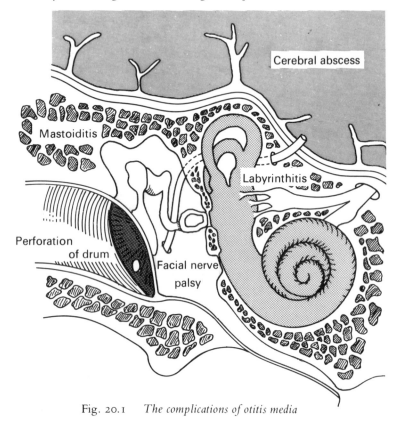

Fig. 20.1   *The complications of otitis media*

Children who have persistantly blocked Eustachian tubes and/or repeated attacks of otitis media are liable to a condition familiarly known as *glue ears*. This arises because the middle ear, being a mucus membrane, normally secretes a small amount of mucus and if this cannot drain it gradually thickens until it takes on the colour and consistency of glue. The main effect this has is to steadily muffle the vibration of the ossicles and make the child gradually deaf, which sometimes presents as learning difficulties at school, and the longer the glue remains the thicker it becomes. The usual treatment is therefore to insert a small plastic cylinder called a *grommet* into the drum to allow the fluid to drain.

Otosclerosis is a genetic disorder of the ossicles of the middle ear, especially the last in the chain, the stapes. The bone first becomes spongy and then hardens ('sclerosis') and cements itself to the oval window beyond, so that vibrations are impeded, especially those of a higher frequency. Another consequence is that the stapedius reflex initially over-reacts, and as the function of this tiny muscle is to act as a 'damper' for loud noise, these are excluded and so speech is heard better against a background of noise ('paracusis').

The hearing loss which ensues is usually bilateral and starts in youth, becoming progressively worse into middle-age at which point it may require treatment with more than just a hearing aid. In women the deafness may suddenly worsen during pregnancy or if they go on the Pill, and as both sexes may experience a little vertigo the condition may be misinterpreted as Meniere's disease. The orthodox treatment involves removal of the stapes and its replacement with a small plastic piston, and this generates substantial improvement in the majority. There is also some evidence that small doses of fluoride and calcium stabilises the bone and helps to halt the deterioration.

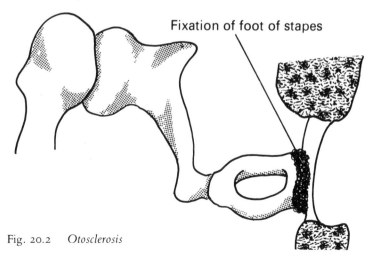

Fixation of foot of stapes

Fig. 20.2   *Otosclerosis*

The Inner Ear

Because the cochlea and the vestibular labyrinth lie so close together and share the vestibulochlear nerve, the symptoms frequently overlap and deafness or tinnitus is often accompanied by vertigo. This is particularly seen in **Meniere's disease**, where there is an increase in the pressure within the labyrinth for reasons which are not clear. The result is periodic distortion of the labyrinth and episodes of vertigo and nausea, tinnitus and a fluctuating hearing loss along with a sense of pressure in the ears. The attacks vary in frequency from one every few months to one a week and may build up over the years, but in between attacks the patient is relatively symptom free.

An individual attack may last from a few hours to several days, effectively confining the patient to bed from the vertigo. As well as these symptoms some sufferers also notice increasing deafness especially for the lower notes, and a degree of tinnitus, and this may eventually remain in between acute attacks. For some reason the fair-skinned, blue-eyed types seem to develop Meniere's disease more readily, usually between the ages of 30–60.

Vertigo

This whirling sensation, often described as giddiness or dizziness, is not an uncommon symptom of other disorders but may occur on its own. *Benign positional vertigo* is the name given to that which occurs only when the head is in a certain position, such as when shaving, seemingly because certain hair cells in the ampulla are easily stimulated. Elderly people are particularly liable to this, but it is usually fatiguable, i.e. it passes off in a few minutes if they maintain the head in that position and then they will be symptom free for several hours.

Labyrinthitis is an occasional consequence of a cold or other viral infection when the labyrinth becomes inflamed and begins to pass false information resulting in severe vertigo which is worse on moving the head. This may lead to extreme nausea and vomiting and last for several days or more, but always clears without serious consequences.

Deafness

It is convenient to divide the causes of deafness into those which arise in the chain of conduction through the outer and middle ear, *conduction deafness*, and those whose origins are in the cochlea or cochlear nerve, *perceptive deafness*. Generally the latter is very much less amenable to treatment owing to its pathology, whereas conductive deafness can at least be helped by a hearing aid if nothing else, as this will amplify sound through the temporal bone itself.

Wax is the commonest reason for conductive deafness, formed by the specialised ceruminous glands in the skin to protect the canal from dirt and water, and which normally clears itself. Some people make large quantities of wax and their ears may require regularly syringing. We have already mentioned such things as otitis media, glue ears and otosclerosis as causes of either muffled hearing or deafness. If one ear is blocked from conducting sound the body is unable to locate the origin of a noise as it relies on the minute difference in timing of the arrival of the sound in the two ears in order to pinpoint the source.

Perceptive deafness is most commonly a result of acoustic trauma, especially in the higher frequencies such as are encountered in many rock bands and in industry. The deterioration is gradual but relentless, and measurement of hearing with audiometry will give an early warning of trouble. Our hearing also deteriorates with age as the cochlear cells degenerate, and it is the peripheral cells, the ones that sense the higer notes, which go first in *presbyacusis* as the deafness of old age is called. This means that when talking to the elderly it is best to speak slowly, clearly and deeply rather than to shout.

Tinnitus

Deafness and tinnitus may go hand in hand, tinnitus being the reaction of the organ of Corti in the cochlea to some kind of stimulus such as inflammation or pressure, while perceptive deafness is the failure to react to that stimulus. Tinnitus is a very common and often distressing disorder, experienced as a continual noise in the head and ranging from a high pitched whistle to a deep booming vibration. As such it is masked by external noise which pushes it into the background, and this is sometimes used as a form of treatment.

The great majority of cases, of which there are about 100,000 in the UK, arise for no obvious reason, although acoustic trauma in the modern world plays a part. Some may arise after a head injury, after certain drugs (particularly streptomycin, an antibiotic sometimes used in TB), after lead poisoning or as one of the symptoms of Meniere's disease or otosclerosis. Arteriosclerosis of the artery supplying the cochlea is thought to cause deterioration of the organ leading to tinnitus in some. There is also a theory that tinnitus results from the minute currents set up in the region by mercury fillings in the teeth, and some have found relief by having their fillings removed.

Bibliography

CHAPTER 1
Fritjof Capra, *The Turning Point*, Penguin Books.
Melvyn Werbach, *Third Line Medicine*, Arkana.
Brian Inglis, *The Diseases of Civilisation*, Paladin.
Ivan Illich, *Medical Nemesis*, Calder & Boyars.
W. G. Spector, *Introduction to General Pathology*, Churchill Livingstone

CHAPTER 2
Staines *et al., Introducing Immunology*, Gower.
Seely *et al., Diet-Related Diseases*, Croom Helm.
Richard Mackarness, *Not All in the Mind*, Pan.

CHAPTER 3
A. P. Ball, *Notes on Infectious Diseases*, Churchill Livingstone.
R. T. Edmond, *Colour Atlas of Infectious Diseases*, Wolfe.

CHAPTER 4
J. L. Burton, *Essentials of Dermatology*, Churchill Livingstone.
G. M. Levene, *Colour Atlas of Dermatology*, Wolfe.

CHAPTER 6
W. Carson Dick, *Introduction to Clinical Rheumatology*, Churchill.
Hamish Watson (ed), *Rheumatology*, MTP Press.

CHAPTER 8
R. Hughes-Jones, *Lecture Notes on Haematology*, Blackwell.
Peter Jones, *Living with Haemophilia*, MTP Press.

CHAPTER 9
M. H. Pappworth, *A Primer of Medicine*, Butterworths.
Hamish Watson (Ed), *Cardiology*, MTP Press.

CHAPTER 11
Donald Lane, *Asthma, The Facts*, Oxford Medical Publications.
Brewis, *Lecture Notes on Respiratory Disease*, Blackwell.

CHAPTER 12
Roy Pounder, *'Doctor, There's something Wrong with my Guts'*, S K & F.

CHAPTER 16
John Day, *The Diabetics Handbook*, Thorsons.

CHAPTER 17
Peter Jeavons, *The Epilepsy Reference Book*, Harper & Row.
A. Burnfield, *Multiple Sclerosis: A Personal Exploration*, Souvenir.
Sir John Walton, *Essentials of Neurology*, Pitman.

CHAPTER 19
Michael Glasspool, *Eyes, their Problems and Treatments*, Martin Druitz.
Hector Bryson Chawla, *Essential Ophthalmology*, Churchill Livingstone

CHAPTER 20
P. D. Bull, *Lecture Notes on Ear, Nose and Throat*, Blackwell.

Glossary of Medical &
Homoeopathic Terms

(Words followed by an asterisk indicate that they are no longer in common usage).

Abscess – A local collection of pus
Achalasia – Inability of organ to relax
Achlorhydria – Absence of acid in the stomach
Acidosis – Excess acidity of the blood
Adenitis – Inflammation of a gland
Adenoma – Benign tumour of glandular tissue
-aemia – Pertaining to the blood
Ague★ – Intermittent fever
Albuminuria – Presence of albumen in the urine
Amaurosis – Transient blindness
Amblyopia – Dimness of vision
Amenorrhoea – Absence of periods
Analgesia – Without pain
Anaphylaxis – Generalised severe allergic reaction
Anasarca★ – Generalised oedema
Angio- – Pertaining to the blood vessels
Ankylosis – Bony fusion
Anorexia – Without appetite
Anoxia – Deficiency of oxygen in the blood
Antibody – Specific substance produced by body in response to
   antigen
Antigen – Substance which to body recognises as not itself
Anuria – Not passing urine
Aphasia – Inability to formulate words in the brain
Aphonia – Inability to convert thoughts into speech
Aphthous – Painful and ulcerated (usually mouth)
Arrhythmia – Abnormal cardiac rhythm
Arthralgia – Painful joints, not necessarily swollen
Arthropathy – Joint disease, not necessarily painful
Ascites – Oedema fluid in the peritoneal cavity
Asthenia★ – Generalised weakness
Ataxia – Unbalanced, staggering

Atopy – Form of hypersensitivity
Atrophy – Withering, loss of size and function
Attenuated – Rendered less harmful

Bacteriuria – Presence of bacteria in urine
Balanitis – Inflammation of glans penis
Balanoposthitis – Same as balanitis, but including foreskin
Benign – Innocent, non life-threatening
Blepharitis – Inflammation of eyelid
Borborygmi – Noises made by peristalsis
Bradycardia – Slow heart beat
Bruit – Noise made by blood in narrowed or tortuous vessel
Bubo★ – Syphilitic gland in the groin
Buccal – Mucus membrane of inside of cheek
Bulimia – Pathologically excessive appetite

Cachexia – Emaciation
Calculus – Stone
Carcinogen – Cancer-producing substance
Casts – Exudates from kidney tubules seen in urine
Catamenia★ – Periods
Cellulitis – Inflammation of connective tissue
Chalazion – Inflamed Meibomian cyst on eyelid
Chemosis – Oedema of conjunctival membrane
Chlorosis★ – Iron deficiency of puberty
Chordee★ – Painful involuntary erection seen in gonorrhoea
Chorea – Involuntary writhing movement
Cicatrix★ – Scar
Climacteric – The changes accompanying the menopause
Clonus/Clonic – Alternating contraction and relaxation of a muscule
Coarctation – Narrowing
Condylomata – Venereal warts
Contagious – Transmitted by touch
Cortex – Outer part or layer of an organ
Crepitation – Cracking sound
Cyanosis – Blue discolouration of blood from increase in CO_2
Cyst – A sac enclosing fluid
-cyte – Type of cell

Dacryocystitis – Inflammation of tear gland
Dementia – Deterioration of mental faculties
Dermographia – Visible reaction of skin to touch or pressure
Dialysis – Separation of substances through a porous membrane
Diaphoresis★ – Increased perspiration
Diastole – Relaxation phase of the heart
Diathesis★ – Constitutional predisposition
Diplopia – Double vision
Diuresis – Passing increased quantity of urine
Dropsy★ – Generalised oedema
Dys- – Under or malfunction in some way
Dysarthria – Difficulty speaking words
Dyslexia – Difficulty reading
Dysmenorrhoea – Painful periods
Dyspepsia – Painful digestion
Dysphasia – Difficulty assembling speech in brain
Dyspnoea – Shortness of breath
Dystrophy – Defective development
Dysuria – Painful urination

Ecchymosis – Large bruise
Eclampsia – Fit associated with pregnancy
Ecthema – Local area of infection of skin which heals with scarring
-ectomy – Removal by surgery
Effusion – Extravasation of fluid into cavity
Embolism – Obstruction of blood vessel by any form of wedge
Emetic – Substance which induces vomiting
Emphysema – Distension of tissues, usually lung
Empyema – Collection of pus in a hollow organ, especially the chest
Endothelium – Internal lining
Enuresis – Urinating in the bed
Epistaxis – Nosebleed
Epithelium – External covering
Eructation – Belching
Erythema – Reddening
Erythism★ – Overexcitability
E.S.R. – Erythrocyte sedimentation rate, a type of blood test

Febricula★ – Short, mild fever

Felon – Inflammation of side of nail

Fibrillation – Irregular heart beat caused by overexcitable myocardium

Fibroma – Benign tumour of fibrous tissue

Fibrosis – The formation of fibrous tissue

Fistula – Pathological connection between two epithelial surfaces

Flatus – Gas in the intestines

Foetor – Offensive odor

Formications★ – Sensation as if ants were crawling over the skin

Furuncle – Boil

Ganglion – Collection of nerve cells outside the CNS/cyst of a joint

Gangrene – Death of tissue, usually from inadequate blood supply

Gingivitis – Inflammation of gums

Gleet★ – Mucoid discharge from the penis

Glossal – Pertaining to the tongue

Glycogen – Form in which carbohydrate is stored in liver and muscles

Goitre – Thyroid swelling

Granuloma – Clusters of cells in chronic inflammation

Gumma – Swelling seen in tertiary syphilis

Haematemesis – Vomiting blood

Haematuria – Passing blood in the urine

Haemolysis – Breakdown of erythrocytes liberating haemo-globin

Haemoptysis – Coughing up blood

Haemostasis – Clotting of the blood

Halitosis – Bad breath

Hemicrania – Headache affecting one side of the head

Hemiparesis – Weakness of one half of the body

Hemiplegia – Paralysis of one half of the body

Hepatomegaly – Enlargement of the liver

Hetero- – Different

Homo- – Same

Hordeolum – Stye
Hydrocoele – Collection of fluid in the scrotum
Hyper- – Excessive
Hypo- – Under, insufficient
Hypochondrium – Area of the abdomen beneath the ribs

Iatrogenic – Doctor-induced
Icterus – Jaundice
Idiopathic – Of unknown origin
Incubus★ – Nightmare
Indurated – Hardened
Infarct – Death of part or whole of an organ from lack of blood
Inter- – Between
Intertrigo – Rash occurring between two surfaces in contact
Ischaemia – Insufficient blood supply to maintain full function
Iso- – Same
-itis – Suffix applied to organ or tissue indicating inflammation

Jactition★ – Extreme restlessness
Jaundice – Excess bile in the blood

Keratitis – Inflammation of the cornea
Kernicterus – Bile deposits in the basal ganglia
Ketonuria – Ketones in the urine
Koilonychia – Spoon-shaped nails
Kyphosis – Hunch-backed

Laparotomy – Operation involving opening the abdominal cavity
Laparoscopy – Inspection of the inside of the abdomen
Lesion – Local pathological change in a tissue
Leuco- – White
Leucocytosis – Increased quantity of leucocytes in the blood
Leucopenia – Decreased quantity of leucocytes in the blood
Lienteric★ – Presence of fatty stools
Lipoma – Benign tumour of fatty tissue
Lumen – Hollow inside of an organ or tube
Lymphoma – Tumour of lymphatic tissue
Lysis – Dissolution

Macro- – Large
Macule – Flat skin lesion
Marasmus – Severe wasting of baby, 'failure to thrive'
Meatus – Canal, opening
Melaena – Passage of dark, digested blood in the stools
Mentagra★ – Barber's itch
Metastasis – Spread of disease from one part of the body to
    another
Micturition – Urination
Micro- – Small
Miliary – Wide dissemination resembling millet seeds
Morphology – Shape
Mural – Pertaining to a wall or surface
Muscae (Volitantes) – Floaters in the eye
Mydriatic – A drug which dilates the pupil
Myeloid – Pertaining to the bone marrow or spinal cord
Myo- – Muscle
Myopic – Short sighted
Myositis – Inflammation of a muscle
Myotic – A drug which constricts the pupil

Naevus – Benign tumour of blood vessels in skin
Nates★ – Buttocks
Necrosis – Death of tissue
Neoplasm – Abnormal new growth in a tissue or organ
Neuralgia – Pain in the distribution of a nerve
Neurasthenia★ – General weakness
Nystagmus – Involuntary rapid tremour of the eyeballs

Oedema – Leakage of fluid into tissues
Oligo- – Insufficient, a few
Oliguria – Passing very small quantities of urine
Omentum – Fatty tissue in abdominal cavity
Onanism★ – Masturbation
Oophoritis – Inflammation of the ovary
Opisthotonous – Arching of the back
Orchitis – Inflammation of the testis
Ortho- – Proper, upright
Orthopnoea – Unable to breath easily when lying flat
-osis – State, condition

Otalgia – Pain in the ear
Otorrhoea – Discharge from the ear
-ostomy – Making an opening
-otomy – Cutting, dividing
Ozaena★ – Discharging nasal ulcer

Papilloedema – Oedema of the optic disc
Papule – Raised skin lesion
Paraplegia – Paralysis of both legs
Paronychia – Inflammation of nail bed, whitlow
Paroxysm – Explosive symptom
Predunculated – Having a stalk
Perinaeum – Area between the legs
Pernio★ – Chilblain
Pes – Foot
Petechiae – Small bruises
Phagodenic★ – Flesh-eating ulcer
Phimosis – Tight foreskin
Phthisis – Tuberculosis
Pleurodynia – Painful intercostal muscles
Plexus – A network
Poly- – Many
Presbyacusis – Deafness of advancing age
Presbyopia – Longsightedness of advancing age
Priapism – Painful, involuntary, sustained erection
Proctitis – Inflammation of the rectum
Prodromal – Transient symptoms preceding the main illness
Purpura – Rash characterised by widespread tiny bruises
Pustule – Small collection of pus under the skin
Pyelitis – Infection of the kidney pelvis
Pyrexia – Fever
Pyrosis★ – Heartburn

Rales – Wheezing sound heard in the chest
Retro- – Behind
Rigor – Severe shivering
Rupia★ – Blistering and scabbing of the skin

Scirrhus – Type of carcinoma characterised by hardness
Sclerosis – Hardening

Splenomegaly – Enlargement of spleen
Serpiginous – Irregularity (of ulcer)
Singultus★ – Hiccup
Sordes – Crusts
Spondylosis – Condition involving the vertebrae
Steatorrhoea – Fatty, undigested stools
Stenosis – Narrowing
Stoma – Aperture, mouth
Strabismus – Squint
Subluxation – Partial dislocation
Suppurate – To form pus
Syncope – Fainting
Syndrome – Collection of symptoms
Synovitis – Inflammation of synovial membrane of joints
Systole – Contraction phase of the heart

Tachy- – Rapid
Tachycardia – Rapid heart beat
Tenesmus – Painful, ineffectual attempt to empty bowel
Tenosynovitis – Inflammation of tendon sheath
Thrombosis – Blood clot
Tinnitus – Ringing in the ears
Torticollis – Spasm of sternomastoid muscle causing stiff neck

Uraemia – Presence of excess urea in the blood
Urticaria – Nettle-rash
Uvea – Area of eye which includes choroid, iris and ciliary body

Varices – Tortuous, dilated veins
Vesicle – Small blister on skin
Viscera – Internal organs
Volvulus – Blockage of the bowel caused by twisting

Whitlow – Infection of the nail bed

INDEX